Lasers in Medical Diagnosis and Therapy

Basics, applications and future prospects

Series in Physics and Engineering in Medicine and Biology

About the Series

Series in Physics and Engineering in Medicine and Biology will allow IPEM to enhance its mission to 'advance physics and engineering applied to medicine and biology for the public good.'

Focusing on key areas including, but not limited to:

- clinical engineering
- diagnostic radiology
- informatics and computing
- magnetic resonance imaging
- nuclear medicine
- physiological measurement
- radiation protection
- radiotherapy
- rehabilitation engineering
- ultrasound and non-ionising radiation.

Lasers in Medical Diagnosis and Therapy

Basics, applications and future prospects

Stephan Wieneke
University of Applied Sciences and Arts HAWK, Göttingen, Germany

Christoph Gerhard
Technical University of Applied Sciences, Wildau, Germany

IOP Publishing, Bristol, UK

ISBN 978-0-7503-1275-2 (ebook)
ISBN 978-0-7503-1277-6 (print)
ISBN 978-0-7503-1276-9 (mobi)

DOI 10.1088/978-0-7503-1275-2

Version: 20180901

IOP Expanding Physics
ISSN 2053-2563 (online)
ISSN 2054-7315 (print)

British Library Cataloguing-in-Publication Data: A catalogue record for this book is available from the British Library.

Published by IOP Publishing, wholly owned by The Institute of Physics, London

IOP Publishing, Temple Circus, Temple Way, Bristol, BS1 6HG, UK

US Office: IOP Publishing, Inc., 190 North Independence Mall West, Suite 601, Philadelphia, PA 19106, USA

This book is dedicated to Anja, Justin Danny, Martina, Benjamin, and Philipp.

Contents

Preface

The capabilities and properties of lasers are often misunderstood and many people take laser irradiation as a generally dangerous phenomenon—a fact which might be due to the distorted image provided by some TV shows and movies. However, lasers are light sources used on a daily basis and a number of consumer goods as well as devices and apparatus used in daily life such as, for example, compact disc players, cash desk scanners, or motion sensors would not work without lasers.

If used carefully, lasers open new possibilities and applications in medicine and in some cases, there are no alternative methods available. Moreover, laser-based approaches can often reduce damage and discomfort after surgical interventions as an alternative to classical methods. In the last decades, lasers have thus become established as essential tools in therapy and surgery, but also in diagnosis and biophotonics and are highly relevant in clinical practice as well as in fundamental and applied research where novel approaches are investigated. Such research is essential and may, in the future, result in the development of laser-based therapy methods for currently non-curable diseases. In the last 30 years, the number of publications containing both the search terms 'laser' and 'medicine' has increased by a factor of approximately 56 from 57 articles in 1986 to 3199 articles in 2017 according to PubMed, the database for medical publications of the National Library of Medicine of the United States of America. This fact shows the increasing relevance of lasers in medical research.

This relevance is also expressed by the rapidly growing demand and market for medical laser sources and systems. According to a forecast published by the business intelligence provider Visiongain in 2015, the world market for medical laser systems will nearly double in the next eight years from a revenue of approximately 500 million dollars in 2017 to approximately 950 million dollars in 2025. The education of skilled personnel in both the development and application of such lasers will thus most likely gain importance in the future.

Against this background, the aim of the present book is to provide an overview of laser applications in medicine for students, lecturers and researchers, mainly in the fields of medicine and surgery, medical engineering and technology, medical physics, ophthalmology, dermatology, laser-based diagnosis as well as biophotonics, but also plastic surgery, laser development, and optical engineering and photonics. It is intended to serve as a textbook for students and lecturers and for the preparation of exams, and thus presents basics, underlying mechanisms, applications and the newest developments of lasers and laser-based diagnosis and therapeutic methods. It also includes a number of exercises and worked examples as well as a formulary and comprehensive chapter summaries in order to point out the most important contents and key information. The subjects covered are the basics of laser sources and medical laser systems including the generation, properties, and guidance of laser irradiation, the interaction mechanisms of laser beams with biological tissue as well as established methods and future prospects of laser diagnosis and therapy.

Göttingen, in February 2018
Stephan Wieneke

Wildau, in February 2018
Christoph Gerhard

Acknowledgements

The authors would like to thank all the people who contributed to the present book for their help during the creation process, especially Jessica Fricchione, Daniel Heatley and Chris Benson from IOP Publishing as well as Christian Ochs, Henrik Werner, and Anna Scheglov from the University of Applied Sciences and Arts in Göttingen.

Author biographies

Stephan Wieneke

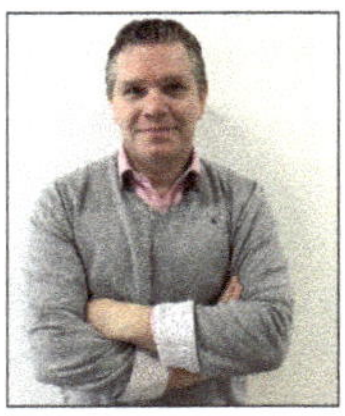

Prof Dr rer nat Stephan Wieneke is a professor for laser-plasma-hybrid technology at the University of Applied Sciences and Arts in Göttingen, Germany, where he has also taught applied laser medicine since 2004. In the last few years, he was also involved in the development and establishment of the new course at this university covering the study of medical engineering.

After his apprenticeship as a physics laboratory assistant he studied physical technology at the University of Applied Sciences and Arts and earned his first diploma degree in 1999. From 1999 to 2008, he worked as a research associate at this university and at the Institute of Mechatronics and Applied Photonics in Göttingen, Germany. During that time, he also studied physics at Clausthal University of Technology in Clausthal–Zellerfeld, Germany and graduated as a physicist with a diploma thesis on carbon dioxide lasers. In 2008, he earned his doctoral degree in physics at Clausthal University. In his thesis, he investigated the generation of far ultraviolet irradiation via laser-pumped *z*-pinch plasmas. From 2009 to 2011, Professor Wieneke was head of the department for laser-plasma-hybrid technology at the Laser Laboratory Göttingen. He subsequently worked as a research associate and lecturer at the University of Applied Sciences and Arts HAWK and at Fraunhofer Institute for Surface Engineering and Thin Films IST, Application Center for Plasma and Photonics in Göttingen, Germany until his appointment as research professor for laser-plasma-hybrid technology in 2013 and subsequent appointment as full professor in 2016.

Professor Wieneke is a member of the German Physical Society. He is the editor of a reference book on laser ablation and has published over 50 articles in optics, laser science and plasma science.

Christoph Gerhard

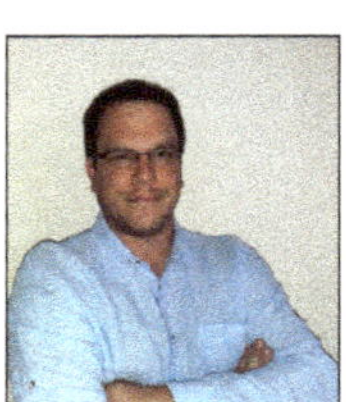

Prof Dr rer nat Christoph Gerhard is a professor for laser and plasma technology at the Technical University of Applied Sciences of Wildau, Germany and a visiting professor for optical system design at the Polytechnic University of Milan, Italy.

After his apprenticeship as an optics technician and a subsequent period as skilled worker and instructor he completed his diploma study in precision manufacturing technology at the University of Applied Sciences and Arts in Göttingen, Germany. In 2006, he prepared his diploma thesis on the development of novel laser sources at the Laboratoire Charles Fabry de l'Institut d'Optique in Orsay, France. For this work, he was awarded the Georg-Simon-Ohm Award by the German Physical Society.

During his work as a product manager for precision optics in industry, he extra-occupationally completed a master's study in optical engineering and photonics at the University of Applied Sciences and Arts. In 2009, he started to work as a technical staff member and research associate at the Bremen Institute for Applied Beam Technology in Bremen, Germany where he finally prepared his master's thesis on optical inline process monitoring of laser-based materials processing techniques. From 2010 to 2016, he worked as the scientific coordinator of the Lower Saxony Innovation Network for Plasma Technology in Göttingen and Clausthal–Zellerfeld, Germany and as a researcher at the Application Center for Plasma and Photonics of the Fraunhofer Institute for Surface Engineering and Thin Films IST in Göttingen, Germany.

In 2014, he earned a doctoral degree in natural sciences and physical technologies at Clausthal University of Technology in Clausthal–Zellerfeld. For his thesis on plasma-assisted laser materials processing he was awarded the Young Talent Award Green Photonics of the Fraunhofer Society in 2015. From 2016 to 2017, he held the position of an adjunct professor for physical technologies at the University of Applied Sciences and Arts.

Professor Gerhard is a member of the German Physical Society and the German Society for Plasma Technology. He has published over 60 papers in the fields of optics and laser and plasma technology and authored two textbooks on the basics of optics and manufacturing of optical components and systems. Moreover, he is the main editor of a reference book on laser ablation.

Chapter 1

Laser basics

This Chapter gives an introduction to the principles of the generation of laser light and the essential underlying laser conditions. The basic setup and components of a laser source as well as the most relevant lasers and laser types used in medicine including the particular properties and fields of application are presented. This includes different solid sate lasers, gas lasers and dye lasers. Finally, important aspects of laser safety and potential primary and secondary risks of laser irradiation are discussed.

1.1 Generation of laser irradiation

It is recorded that after the presentation of the very first operating laser source in August 1960 two pioneers of laser development, Theodore Maiman and Arthur Schawlow, stated that 'the laser is a solution in search of a problem'. Obviously, a number of extremely different problems, or rather challenges and applications, have been identified and nowadays, lasers are essential components in modern technology, research and medicine. The reason for the singular properties of laser irradiation is hidden in its acronym: **LASER** = **L**ight **A**mplification by **S**timulated **E**mission of **R**adiation. Stimulated emission of light, the basic physical mechanism of laser sources, was first theoretically described by Albert Einstein in 1916. Twelve years later, in 1928, this type of emission was demonstrated experimentally by Rudolf Ladenburg. On the basis of this work, the precursor of lasers, the **MASER** (= **M**icrowave **A**mplification by **S**timulated **E**mission of **R**adiation) was realised by Nikolay Basov, Aleksandr Prokhorov and Charles Townes in 1954. Six years later, the first laser, a ruby laser, was then presented by Theodore Maiman and Charles Asawa. Thenceforward, the development of laser sources and laser-based processes were amongst the most rapidly growing fields in fundamental and applied research and still are. In 1962, merely two years after the presentation of Maiman's ruby laser, the first diode laser was developed and in 1964, a new solid state laser, the

doi:10.1088/978-0-7503-1275-2ch1

neodymium-doped yttrium aluminium garnet laser, and the first gas laser, a carbon dioxide laser, were invented. Nowadays, these two lasers are amongst the most important laser sources in research, industry and medicine. In paricular, the development and improvement of lasers providing short pulses in the 1980s and the invention of laser amplifiers has opened a large number of new fields of applications. However, the basic physical mechanisms and conditions for the generation of laser irradiation have not changed since its first description in 1916. These mechanisms and conditions, as well as the setup of laser sources commonly used for medical applications, are presented in the following sections.

1.1.1 The laser principle and conditions

As expressed by its acronym, laser irradiation is generated by first, stimulated emission of radiation and second, amplification of the emitted light where the process of stimulated emission is the basic mechanism. It significantly differs from spontaneous emission, the driving force for the generation of light in classical light sources such as the Sun or lamps. Both spontaneous emission and stimulated emission result from a so-called population inversion which comes off as follows: taking the Rutherford–Bohr model of an atom and the position of its electrons in thermodynamic equilibrium as a basis, more electrons are found on lower electron paths, i.e. at lower energy levels close to the atom core and fewer electrons are situated on higher electron paths and higher energy levels, respectively. The number of electrons N_x at any energy level x of an atom can then be determined on the basis of the Boltzmann distribution, given by

$$N_x = N_1 \cdot e^{-\frac{E_x}{k_B \cdot T}} \tag{1.1}$$

Here, N_1 is the number of electrons in the ground state E_1, k_B is the Boltzmann constant[1] and T is the absolute temperature. For the generation of light, this distribution has to be inverted, i.e. electrons have to be excited from a lower energy level to a higher one by introducing external energy to the atom. In the case of artificial light generation (and especially in laser technology), such introduction of energy is referred to as pumping. Pumping of electrons from a lower ground level to a higher state finally results in a population inversion, as shown in figure 1.1.

After a short lifetime at such a higher energy level, the electron spontaneously falls back to its initial (ground) state in order to compensate the excited state of the atom. At the same time, a light wave is emitted, as shown in figure 1.2.

The energy E released in the course of this de-excitation process corresponds to the difference in energy between the higher (E_2) and the lower (E_1) energy level. It corresponds to the photon energy E_{photon} of the light wave emitted by spontaneous emission, given by

[1] The Boltzmann constant is $k_B = 1.38 \cdot 10^{-23}$ J K^{-1}.

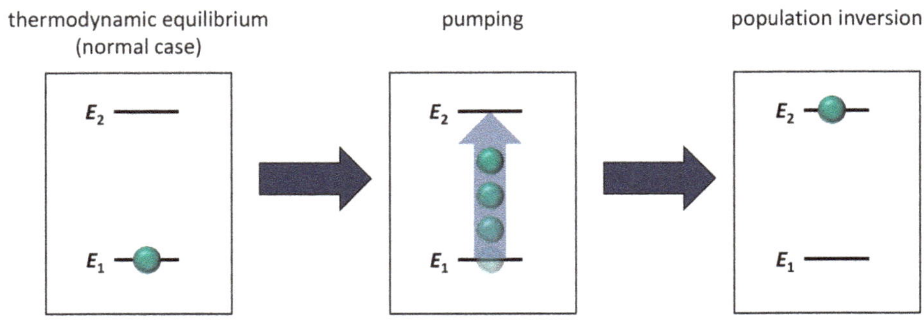

Figure 1.1. Visualisation of the formation of population inversion of an electron; the electron which populates a lower energy level E_1 in an atom (left) is pumped to a higher level E_2 by external energy (middle), finally leading to population inversion (right).

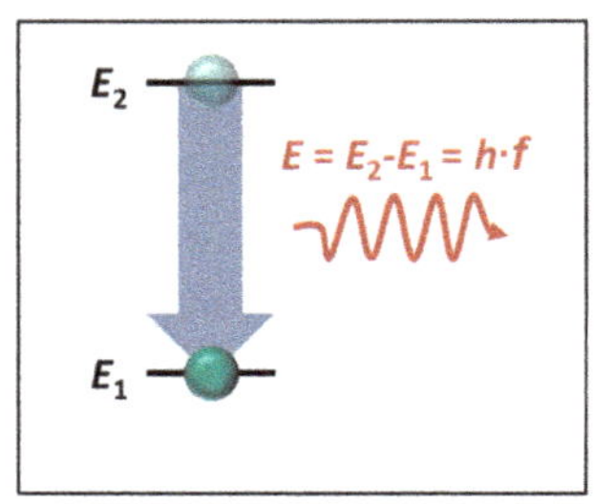

Figure 1.2. Spontaneous emission of light during de-excitation of an electron from a higher energy level E_2 to its ground state E_1 where the difference of both energy levels is the energy E of the emitted light.

$$E_{\text{photon}} = h \cdot f \tag{1.2}$$

with h being Planck's constant[2] and f being the frequency of the emitted light wave. Consequently, the wavelength λ of the emitted light, given by

$$\lambda = \frac{c_0}{f} = \frac{c_0 \cdot h}{E_2 - E_1} \tag{1.3}$$

directly follows from the difference in energy between the upper excited energy level E_2 and the ground state E_1. It thus mainly depends on the atom or medium where emission takes place. Note that the parameter c_0 in equation (1.3) is the speed of light in a vacuum[3]. Metaphorically speaking, such spontaneous emission of light is the ignition spark of stimulated emission since the very first, initial light wave which starts the process of stimulated emission originates from spontaneous emission. As shown in figure 1.3, the initial light wave causes the stimulated de-excitation of an electron which was pumped to a higher energy level. During de-excitation, this electron emits a further, duplicated light wave. As a result, the light wave emitted in

[2] Planck's constant is $h = 6.626 \cdot 10^{-34}$ m^2 kg s^{-1}.
[3] The speed of light in vacuum is $c_0 = 3 \cdot 10^8$ m s^{-1}.

the course of this process features the same photon energy and wavelength, respectively, as the incident wave. Laser irradiation is thus almost monochromatic[4].

Further, there is no phase retardation of both waves, the incident and the duplicated one. In a subsequent avalanche process, a multitude of such identical waves is generated. All these light waves are coherent and thus superimpose in phase, giving rise to constructive interference. As a consequence of such interference and the accompanying successive accumulation of the particular intensities of duplicated waves, the light is amplified during each round trip within the laser resonator and the laser active gain medium, respectively. The principle of this effect which finally gives the actual laser operation is shown in figure 1.4.

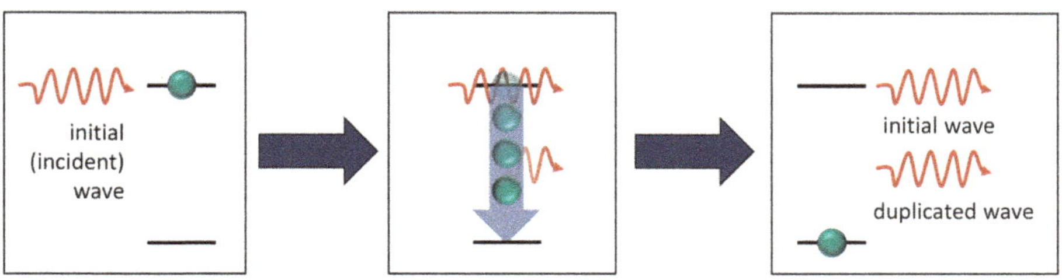

Figure 1.3. Stimulated emission of light where de-excitation of an electron is induced by an initial, incident light wave (left); the new light wave generated in the course of such de-excitation (middle) is a duplicate of the initial wave (right).

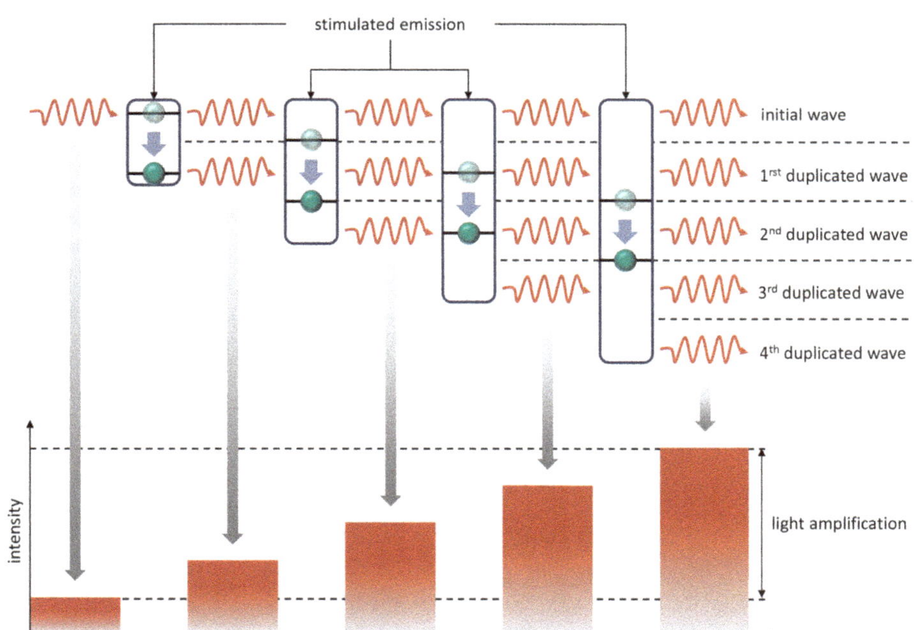

Figure 1.4. Principle of light amplification by constructive interference of coherent light waves emitted by stimulated emission.

[4] In reality, laser irradiation features a certain spectral linewidth due to natural line broadening mechanisms.

One has to consider that for such laser operation two conditions, the so-called laser conditions, have to be fulfilled:

- for the generation of laser light, population inversion must be realised initially
- when passing through a laser resonator, the amplification of light by constructive interference must be higher than losses of light.

The second laser condition addresses the actual and physical setup of a laser source. The losses mentioned there could arise from absorption or scattering within optical components of a laser setup or be due to reflection and scattering at the surface of such components. The essential elements and optical components of laser resonators and sources are introduced in more detail in the following section.

1.1.2 Setup of laser sources

In order to obtain light amplification via constructive interference, a standing light wave has to be realised. This is achieved by one of the most essential parts of a laser setup, the laser resonator or laser cavity. Such a resonator basically consists of two opposite mirrors, a highly reflective end mirror and a partially reflective output mirror, as shown in figure 1.5.

The light emitted by the laser active medium forms a standing wave, also referred to as longitudinal mode, if the so-called resonator condition, given by

$$\lambda = \frac{2 \cdot l_r}{N} \tag{1.4}$$

is fulfilled. Here, λ is the wavelength of the laser light, l_r is the length of the laser resonator, i.e. the distance between the two mirrors, and N is an integer. Thus, the double resonator length must correspond to an integral multiple of the laser wavelength. Once this condition is fulfilled, a standing light wave is formed between the mirrors and a portion of light is coupled out by the output mirror. In order to achieve stimulated emission and constructive interference, the laser active medium, also known as the gain medium, is placed within the resonator. Population inversion

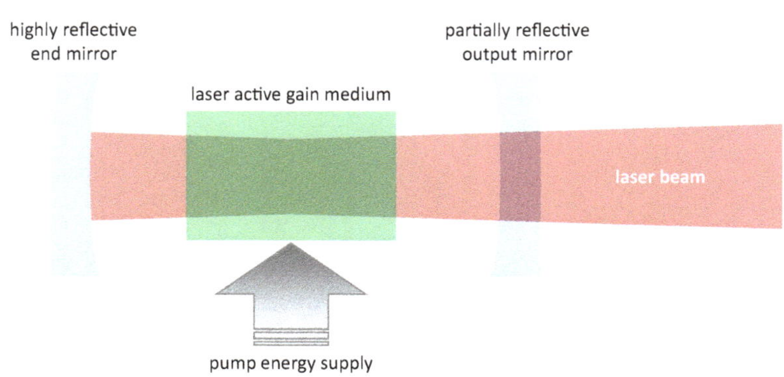

Figure 1.5. Scheme of a basic laser setup consisting of two mirrors which form the laser resonator, the laser active gain medium and a pump energy supply.

within the laser active gain medium is obtained by introducing an external energy supply in order to pump electrons from the ground state to an upper, excited state. This can be realised either electrically by applying a high voltage-based electric discharge as is usually required in the case of gaseous laser active gain media and semiconductors or optically, e.g. by flash lamps or incident laser irradiation as is typically applied for classical crystalline solid state gain media. To summarise, the essential components of a laser source are:

- the laser resonator, basically consisting of two mirrors
- the laser active gain medium, and
- a pump energy supply.

However, modern laser sources contain a number of further optical elements or closed electro-optical systems, e.g. for the generation of short laser pulses. Once the laser operation has started such a simple basic laser setup as described above emits continuous laser irradiation (continuous wave, cw) with a certain average output power. But for many applications in medicine and biophotonics, short pulses with pulse durations in the nanosecond (e.g. for plasma-mediated ablation of tissue), picosecond (e.g. for the detection of short-lived fluorophores) or even femtosecond (e.g. for laser assisted *in situ* keratomileusis) range are required. The main advantages of short laser pulses in comparison to continuous wave laser irradiation are the achievable high pulse energies and pulse peak powers, respectively, and the short time of interaction of laser irradiation with tissue, resulting in a reduction of thermal impact. Short laser pulses are generated by placing an active or passive switch within the laser resonator. A well-established active switch is the so-called Pockels cell which basically consists of a crystal, a high-voltage power supply and a polariser. When exposed to high voltage, the polarisation of laser light travelling through the crystal is turned by a voltage-dependent value as a result of the electro-optical effect. After passing the crystal, laser light is then deflected towards a beam dump by the polariser if the polarisation fits well the orientation of the polariser; the deflected portion of light is thus not sent to the laser resonator's output mirror. Such a Pockels cell allows generating short pulses where the pulse duration and the pulse repetition rate can be adjusted by the high voltage applied to the crystal. However, this type of optical switch is limited by the circuit time of the used power supply. Consequently, the pulse duration is quite long, i.e. in the range of a number of microseconds or nanoseconds. Shorter laser pulses are thus realised by passive switches and mainly by so-called saturable absorbers[5].

There are a number of different types of saturable absorbers and basically, the principle of this type of optical switch can be explained as follows: within a laser resonator, all longitudinal laser modes which fulfil the resonator condition according to equation (1.4) can oscillate. Some of these modes may interfere arbitrarily and

[5] Saturable absorbers can work as a transmissive or reflective device. In the latter case, such a saturable absorber consists of several stacked thin layers made of different semiconducting materials. In contrast, transparent saturable absorbers such as for example quadratic polarisation switchers are mainly based on nonlinear optical effects.

form a short pulse with a much higher peak energy than the other oscillating modes. The oscillation of this single pulse is then further supported by a saturable absorber mirror. Such a mirror, usually the end mirror of the resonator, absorbs laser irradiation at low power and energy, respectively, but reflects laser irradiation which exceeds a certain saturation intensity. The randomly formed laser pulse is thus selected and reflected, it then passes the laser active medium and is further amplified. The duration of this pulse follows from the relaxation time of the saturable absorber which typically amounts to a number of picoseconds. However, shorter pulses in the femtosecond and even attosecond range can be realised nowadays. For this purpose, the picosecond laser pulse generated as described above is further compressed by suitable optics such as an arrangement of dispersion prisms within the laser resonator. Such prisms are further components which increase the losses. According to the second laser condition, this has to be compensated by a higher gain in comparison to a simple continuous wave laser.

As a consequence of the number of optical components involved and the accompanying losses as well as the partially low conversion efficiency of some active devices, the output power or energy of laser resonators may be insufficient for the selected applications. In this case, laser irradiation is amplified by optical amplifiers which are arranged outside the actual laser resonator. A laser amplifier could be referred to as a second laser setup without any resonator. It thus consists of a further laser active gain medium, i.e. the same as is found within the resonator, which is pumped in order to generate population inversion. Stimulated emission from this amplifier medium then occurs when an incident laser beam passes through the medium and initiates stimulated emission. This incident laser beam, coming from the laser resonator, is consequently amplified in terms of power or energy. Modern amplifiers contain several amplification stages and a large variety of different setups are in hand: in sequential amplifiers, a number of single amplifiers are arranged in series, whereas the laser beam passes through one and the same laser active gain medium several times in so-called multi-pass amplifier systems. Apart from the generation of short laser pulses and the amplification of laser irradiation, the possibility of changing a laser source's emission wavelength is of great practical interest and can be achieved as follows: laser irradiation of high intensity (in the case of continuous wave laser) or fluence (in the case of pulsed lasers) can provoke nonlinear optical effects when passing through suitable media. One nonlinear optical effect is the formation of the second harmonic of the incident laser beam. That means that the fundamental laser beam's frequency, which is directly related to its wavelength, is doubled. As a result, the wavelength is halved. The most common example for the technical application of this effect is the Nd:YAG solid state laser where the fundamental wavelength as emitted by the gain medium is 1064 nm (i.e. near infrared radiation). After frequency doubling, laser irradiation at a wavelength of 532 nm (i.e. green light) is generated. This process can be repeated a number of further times, where usually the third and fourth harmonic can be generated. Referring to Nd:YAG lasers, this corresponds to a wavelength of 355 nm (i.e. near ultraviolet, UV-A) and 266 nm (i.e. far ultraviolet, UV-C), respectively. Since such processes are subject to a limited conversion efficiency, fifth or even sixth harmonic generation are not feasible in practice.

1.2 Lasers and laser types used in medicine

Maiman and Schawlow's doubts ('The laser is a solution in search of a problem.') were dispelled merely two years later. In 1963, several quite different laser applications such as laser-based micromachining of diaphragms with inner diameters in the range of a number of microns or laser-induced breakdown spectroscopy for material analysis were reported in the literature. And, very soon after the invention and realisation of the laser, laser sources were also used for medical purposes such as for example the treatment of tissue. The laser wavelengths used here vary from the ultraviolet to the far infrared spectral range. For instance, argon fluoride (ArF) excimer lasers, where the wavelength is 193 nm, are used in ophthalmology or carbon dioxide (CO_2) lasers with an emission wavelength of 10.6 μm are applied in surgery for cutting and drilling tissue and bones. Figure 1.6 gives an overview on the entire spectrum of laser systems used in medicine.

The classification of laser types is usually based on the state of aggregation of the particular laser active gain medium. The main groups of lasers are thus solid state lasers, gas lasers and dye lasers, where the gain medium of the latter type of laser is a liquid. Following this classification, the most important laser sources used in medicine are presented in more detail in the following sections.

1.2.1 Solid state lasers

The neodymium–YAG laser

Nowadays, the neodymium-doped yttrium aluminium garnet (Nd:YAG) laser is the most important and well-established solid state laser and is used in a number of different fields of application such as materials processing, metrology and laser medicine. This type of laser source stands out due to its simple, compact and robust setup and its high mean laser power. Depending on the particularly applied type of pumping and excitation, either by flash lamps or laser diodes, its degree of efficiency amounts to approximately 2–5%. Generally, the laser active medium used in such lasers, the neodymium Nd^{3+} ion, can be embedded and operated in different host crystals or glasses. However, the yttrium aluminium garnet ($Y_3Al_5O_{12}$, usually

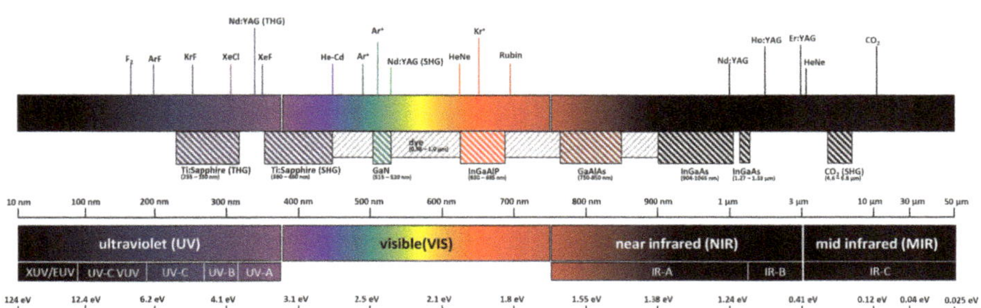

Figure 1.6. Overview of medical laser systems.

abbreviated YAG) crystal system has turned out to be the most suitable one due to the comparable size of neodymium ions and yttrium ions which are replaced by the actual laser active Nd^{3+} ions in the course of the doping process during crystal growth. The concentration of these ions within the YAG host crystal typically amounts to about 1.5 volume per cent. At present, Nd:YAG crystals with a maximum length of 150 mm can be produced where crystal rods with a diameter of approximately 3–7 mm and a length of about 90–150 mm are usually used for laser sources. As shown in figure 1.7, Nd:YAG lasers are four-level lasers.

Here, the energy levels and the laser transition of Nd:YAG is shown where the Nd^{3+} ions are found in the ground state initially. As a consequence of absorption of incident pumping light provided by flash lamps or pumping laser diodes, these ions take an excited state in the excitation bands (2) and the upper metastable and long-lasting laser level (3) is populated due to fast and radiationless transitions. Light emission at a wavelength of 1064 nm (i.e. near infrared light) then follows from the population inversion between the transition of the third and fourth level where some commercially available Nd:YAG lasers also generate radiation at a wavelength of 1320 nm (transition of level (3) to (4′)). Subsequent frequency conversion using nonlinear phenomena in suitable media such as potassium titanyl phosphate ($KTiOPO_4$, usually abbreviated KTP) further allows the generation of shorter wavelengths. For the fundamental Nd:YAG wavelength of 1064 nm, visible green laser light at a wavelength of 532 nm is generated by such a frequency conversion of the second harmonic, whereas the third and fourth harmonic feature a wavelength of 355 nm and 266 nm, respectively, as introduced in section 1.1.2

In practice, pumping of the laser active transition is usually realised using inert gas (e.g. krypton or xenon) arc discharge flash lamps. Such lamps feature emission bands in the range of 500–900 nm which conform quite well to the pump levels. Here, the total efficiency amounts to approximately 2%. The use of laser diodes with an emission wavelength of 805–808 nm as pump source allows increasing the efficiency up to approximately 15% at an output power of 10–15 W.

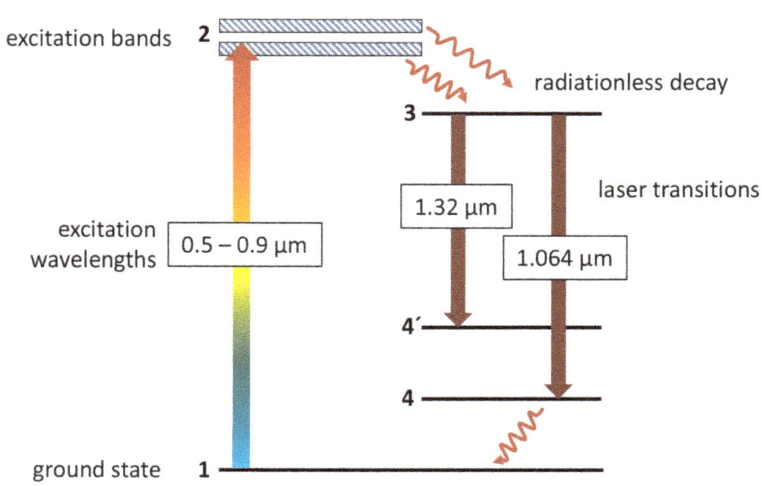

Figure 1.7. Energy levels and laser transition of the four-level laser gain medium Nd:YAG.

Properties, parameters and characteristics

- Laser active gain medium: YAG-crystal, doped with the actual laser active neodymium ion.
- Emission wavelength: 1064 nm.
- Efficiency factor: typically 1–2% for flash lamp-pumped systems and up to 15% for diode-pumped systems (at 10–15 W).
- Pulsed or continuous wave (cw) operation possible.
- Typical pulse duration: 5–20 ns.
- Guidance by fibres possible.
- Simple, compact and robust setup.
- Penetration depth into tissue: approximately 2–8 μm.

Applications in medicine

- Continuous wave (cw) laser for surgical applications such as cutting and drilling [1–3].
- Continuous wave (cw) laser for laser-induced interstitial[6] thermotherapy[7] (LITT), [4–7].
- Long-pulse laser for dermatological applications such as bleaching and dentine sealing [8, 9].
- Q-switched, pulsed laser for laser-induced shock-wave lithotripsy (LISL) or the removal of tattoos [10, 11].

The holmium–YAG laser

The emission wavelength of holmium–YAG (Ho:YAG) lasers is 2.08 μm, i.e. between the emission wavelength of Nd:YAG lasers and carbon dioxide (CO_2) lasers. Such irradiation is relatively strongly absorbed by tissue water where the absorption coefficient is about ten times lower in comparison to CO_2 laser irradiation. As a consequence, the size of the coagulation zone is also found in between the size of coagulation zones resulting from Nd:YAG laser or CO_2 laser irradiation. Holmium–YAG lasers thus fill an intermediary position between pure coagulation and cutting lasers. They can be driven by flash lamps or pump diodes and be operated either in continuous wave or pulsed mode. In the latter case, holmium–YAG lasers provide mean output powers of 30–40 W at pulse durations from 200 to 600 μs, pulse energies from 0.2 to 3.5 J and repetition rates up to 50 Hz. The most efficient medium for this type of solid state laser is chromium, thulium, holmium doped yttrium aluminium garnet (Cr,Tm,Ho:YAG), schematically shown in figure 1.8.

Here, the incident pumping light is either absorbed by the broad absorption band between the A_2 state and the T_2 state of chromium ions at wavelengths from 420 to 600 nm or directly absorbed by energy levels of the thulium ions (Tm^{3+}) from the $^3H_6$ state to the $^3F_4$ state in the case of diode-pumped systems. Radiationless energy transfer occurs from all excited states to the $^3F_4$ energy level of the Tm^{3+} ion.

[6] Interstitial = within the interstitial tissue.

[7] Thermotherapy is also referred to as heat therapy.

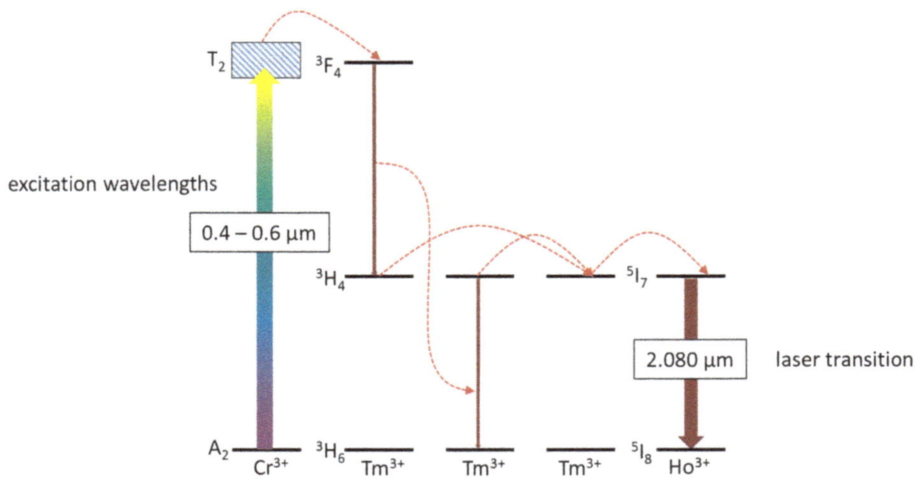

Figure 1.8. Scheme of the Cr,Tm,Ho:YAG laser system (adapted from [12]).

Highly-excited Tm^{3+} ions are de-activated from the $^3F_4$ to the $^3H_4$ energy level. The difference in energy of these two levels corresponds well to the difference in energy of the low-energetic $^3H_6$ and $^3H_4$ level of the Tm^{3+} ion. As a consequence, the resonant energy transfer of a de-activated Tm^{3+} ion to a neighbouring Tm^{3+} ion becomes highly probable. This leads to a so-called cross-relaxation, i.e. the excitation of a thulium ion from the lower $^3H_6$ level to the upper $^3H_4$ level. As a result of such a cross-relaxation process, two Tm^{3+} ions can now be excited to the $^3H_4$ level by a single pumping photon. Due to this resonant energy process, the excitation energy of the $^3H_4$ level travels between neighbouring Th^{3+} ions. As soon as one ion is reached, the energy can be transferred without any emission of radiation to the quasi-resonant higher laser level $^5I_7$ of the holmium ion (Ho^{3+}). Laser irradiation is then emitted during excitation of the Ho^{3+} ion to its lower laser level $^5I_8$, which is quite close to the ground state and thus features a high population density at ambient conditions. Thus, a holmium laser system can be referred to as a quasi-three-level laser system when operated at ambient temperature. As a consequence, high excitation energy becomes necessary for obtaining sufficient population inversion.

Properties, parameters and characteristics

- Laser active gain medium: YAG-crystal, doped with the actual laser active holmium ion as well as chromium and thulium.
- Emission wavelength: 2.06 µm.
- Efficiency factor: typically 3%.
- Pulsed or continuous wave (cw) operation possible.
- Typical pulse duration: 150–800 µs.
- Average output power approximately 30–40 W (up to 200 W possible).
- Penetration depth into tissue: approximately 2–8 mm.

Applications in medicine

- Refractive surgery[8] in ophthalmology [13, 14].
- Treatment of benign prostatic hyperplasia[9](BPH) in urology, [15, 16].
- Fragmentation of vesical calculus[10] [17–19].
- Vaporisation of tissue.

The erbium–YAG laser

For the realisation of erbium–YAG (Er:YAG) lasers, yttrium aluminium garnet crystals are doped with erbium ions at relatively high concentration, i.e. approximately 50%. The wavelength of the resulting laser irradiation amounts to 2.94 μm. When using other crystals as host medium for the actual laser active erbium ion and adding further dopants, this wavelength can be reduced to 2.80 μm (Cr:Er:YSGG[11]), 2.78 μm (Er:YSGG), or 2.64 μm (Cr:Tm:Er:YAG). Due to the complex scheme of the energy levels of erbium[12], as shown in figure 1.9, such lasers can exclusively be operated in the pulsed regime.

As an example, pulsed Er:YAG lasers with pulse durations in the range from 50 to 500 μs exhibit an average output power of around 30 W at a pulse repetition rate of 50–100 Hz. The degree of efficiency of such lasers is 1–2%. In practice and clinical applications, beam guidance of Er:YAG laser beams is usually achieved by mirror-based jointed arms or optical fibres made of germanium oxide.

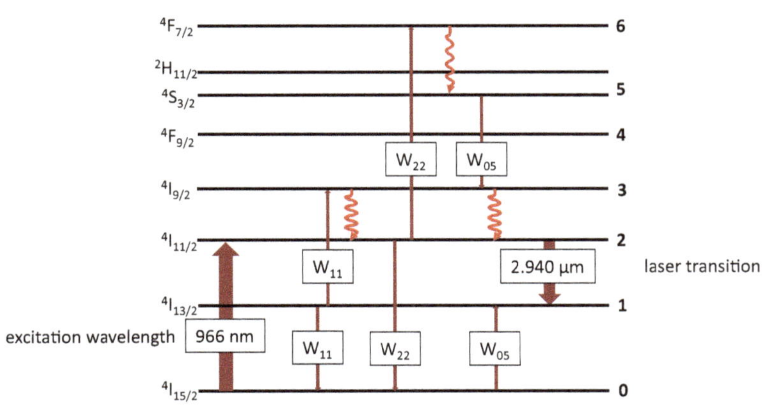

Figure 1.9. Scheme of the erbium–YAG laser system.

[8] The modification of the eye's refractive power by any surgical intervention is referred to as refractive surgery.

[9] Benign prostatic hyperplasia is a noncancerous enlargement of the prostate and is thus also referred to as prostate enlargement.

[10] I.e. bladder stones.

[11] YSSG = yttrium scandium gallium garnet.

[12] Here, energy-transfer-upconversion and cross-relaxation processes take place.

Properties, parameters and characteristics

- Laser active gain medium: YAG-crystal, doped with the actual laser active erbium ion.
- Emission wavelength: 2.94 μm.
- Efficiency factor: typically 1–2%
- Exclusively pulsed operation possible.
- Typical pulse duration: 50–500 μs.
- Highest absorption in water, where the optical penetration depth amounts to a number of microns (1–5 μm).

Applications in medicine

- Removal of soft and hard tissue (due to the high absorption in water) [20–22].
- Dermatological applications for the removal of superficial skin alterations such as verrucas [23].
- Different applications in dentistry and invasive surgery [24, 25].

The alexandrite laser

The laser gain medium of alexandrite (Cr^{3+}:$BeAl_2O_4$) lasers is an alexandrite crystal doped with chromium ions (Cr^{3+}). The eponymous gemstone alexandrite is also known as chrysoberyl, i.e. an aluminate of beryllium with the total formula $BeAl_2O_4$. Such lasers are tunable and can be operated at wavelengths in the range from 700 to 800 nm where the most relevant emission wavelength is 750 nm. One has to consider that in contrast to Nd:YAG lasers, alexandrite lasers are not four-level lasers, but are operated in a quasi-four-level regime, as shown in figure 1.10. This quasi-four-level scheme exhibits a degenerate ground state, $^4A_2$, different excitation states and a multiple degenerate upper laser level. It can thus be compared to an actual three-level system, but exhibits a virtual vibration state which is found above the ground state and thus acts as a fourth (intermediate) energy level. As a consequence, alexandrite lasers can be referred to as quasi-four-level laser systems

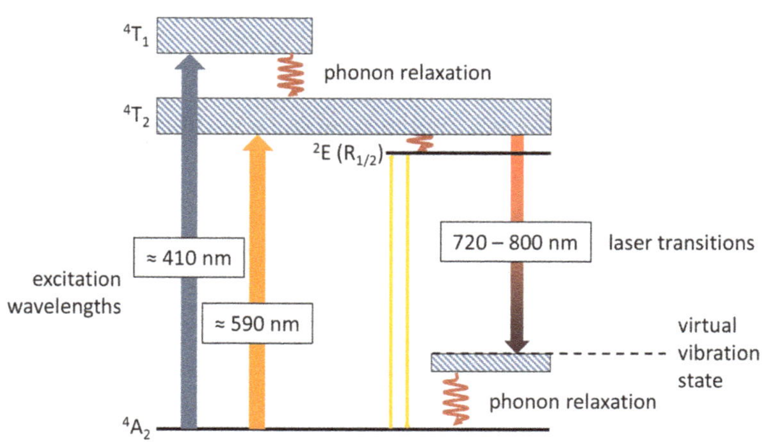

Figure 1.10. Energy levels and laser transition of the quasi-four-level alexandrite laser.

with low lasing threshold[13]. The alexandrite laser, with its large spot size and high repetition rate has now usurped the role of the ruby laser. It is the fastest, most widely used, laser for hair removal and is suitable for rapid treatment of large body areas. Alexandrite lasers can significantly lighten or remove many tattoo inks, and are especially effective for removing green and black inks. Tattoo ink is removed by using a specific wavelength, which passes through the skin but is absorbed by the ink. Alexandrite lasers are also used for treating kidney stones and require very little maintenance and are unlikely to harm the patient.

Properties, parameters and characteristics

- Laser active gain medium: alexandrite (chrysoberyl) crystal, doped with chromium.
- Emission wavelengths: 700–800 nm.
- Efficiency factor: typically 1%.
- Pulsed or continuous wave (cw) operation possible.
- First commercially available tuneable laser.
- High pulse energy possible (up to 3 J).

Applications in medicine

- Disintegration of melanin-containing structures[14] as well as treatment of pigmented moles in dermatology.
- Fragmentation of vesical calculus [26].
- Removal of tattoos [27, 28].
- Laser epilation[15] as well as treatment of pigmented moles in dermatology [29, 30].

The ruby laser

The ruby (Cr^{3+}:Al_2O_3) laser was the first operable laser source, presented by Maiman and Asawa in 1960. Since this laser type is a three-level system, more than 50% of ions have to be excited in order to obtain population inversion and laser operation, respectively. Excitation is accomplished by flash lamps; ruby lasers are thus generally pulsed laser systems and modern ruby lasers can reach pulse energies up to 20 J. The same as for alexandrite lasers, the actual laser active medium of ruby lasers is the chromium ion Cr^{3+} which replaces aluminium ions (Al^{3+}) within the host crystal ruby[16] where the concentration of chromium ions is 0.05 at%. Optical pumping of this laser gain medium results in population inversion from the ground state $^4A_2$ to the excited states $^4F_1$ and $^4F_2$, respectively, of the chromium ion.

[13] The low lasing threshold of alexandrite lasers is due to the fact that classical population inversion of energy levels is not mandatory for laser operation as a result of the presence of vibrational transitions.

[14] Alexandrite laser irradiation features a wavelength of 700–800 nm and is thus mainly absorbed by melanin, i.e. natural pigments, and dyes but not by blood. This allows the selective disintegration of such laser irradiation-absorbing substances and pigments.

[15] I.e. the laser-based removal of body hair.

[16] Ruby is the red-coloured variety of corundum, i.e. the crystalline form of aluminium oxide (Al_2O_3).

As shown in figure 1.11, suitable pump wavelengths are 410 and 560 nm where ruby crystals feature high absorption.

After pumping a fast radiationless decay from the excited states $^4F_1$ and $^4F_2$ to the upper laser level E_2, a metastable level occurs. Laser light is then emitted as a result of the de-excitation from this level to the ground state $^4A_2$. Since the metastable level E_2 consists of two neighbouring levels which slightly differ in terms of energy, the emitted laser light can principally feature two different wavelengths, either 694.3 nm or 692.7 nm. Usually, ruby lasers are operated at an emission wavelength of 694.3 nm. Due to such laser emission in the visible spectral range, guidance of ruby laser beams can be realised with classical refractive optical elements and fibres, but also mirror-based jointed arms are often used in clinical applications.

Properties, parameters and characteristics

- Laser active gain medium: ruby crystal, doped with the actual laser active chromium ion.
- Emission wavelength: 694.3 nm (typical) or 692.7 nm.
- Exclusively pulsed operation possible.
- First operable laser source.

Applications in medicine

- Dermatology (compare applications of alexandrite lasers listed).
- Removal of dark (e.g. black or blue) tattoos [31–33].
- Laser epilation [34].

The titanium sapphire laser

The laser active medium of titanium sapphire (Ti^{3+}:Al_2O_3, usually abbreviated Ti: sapphire or TiSa) lasers is the titanium ion Ti^{3+} which replaces aluminium ions (Al^{3+}) in the host crystal sapphire (Al_2O_3). This crystal can efficiently be pumped at any wavelength in the range from 400 to 600 nm where maximum absorption is found

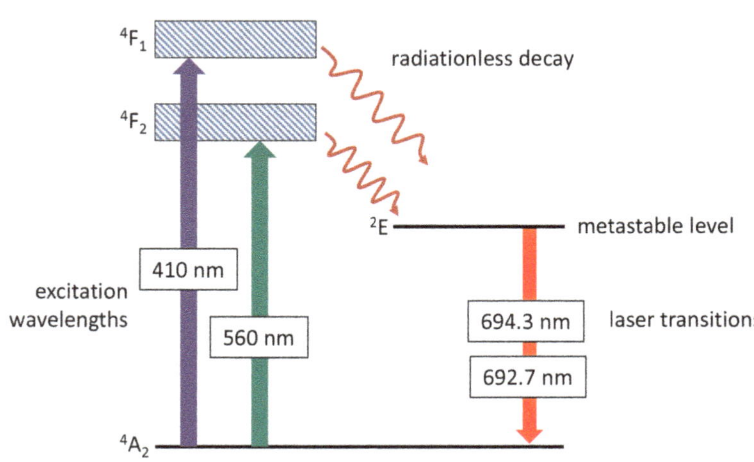

Figure 1.11. Scheme of a ruby laser gain medium including the relevant transitions.

at 490 nm. Since the lifetime of the excited upper laser level is comparatively short, Ti-sapphire lasers are pumped by the second harmonic of pulsed Nd:YAG laser irradiation at 532 nm. Principally, titanium sapphire crystals exhibit a broad fluorescence band, such laser systems are thus tuneable and can provide laser irradiation in the wavelength range from 660 to 1160nm where the maximum intensity is found at approximately 800 nm. Another special feature of Ti:sapphire lasers is the possibility of the generation of ultra-short laser pulses with pulse durations in the range of some tens to hundreds of femtoseconds and at high pulse repetition rates of up to 100 MHz. This allows the realisation of high-power laser sources[17].

Properties, parameters and characteristics

- Laser active gain medium: sapphire crystal, doped with titanium.
- Emission wavelengths: 660–1160 nm, maximum intensity at approximately 800 nm.
- Pulsed or continuous wave (cw) operation possible.
- Very short laser pulse duration possible (down to approximately 4 fs).
- High laser power possible (up to 300 TW).

Applications in medicine

- Two-photon-excitation in microscopy for biophotonics [35, 36].
- Laser assisted *in situ* keratomileusis (LASIK)[18] in ophthalmology [37].

The diode laser

The diode laser, usually also referred to as semiconductor laser, was first presented in 1962. Since that time, it has gained notable importance in a number of fields of application and especially in telecommunications and laser medicine. Its laser active gain medium is a semiconductor which is doped with foreign atoms in order to modify the electrical properties of the basic semiconductor selectively. In the course of this doping process, foreign atoms, the so-called dopants, enter the semiconductor due to diffusion processes and an n-type region and a p-type region are realised within the semiconductor. The first region results in the case of dopants which are capable of delivering electrons (i.e. an n-doping with donators). In contrast, positively-charged defects, also referred to as holes, are produced within the semiconductor if the dopant is able to bond free electrons (i.e. a p-doping with acceptors). Since both regions are directly contacted, an intermediate zone, known as the p–n junction, with a valence-conduction band gap is formed and the Fermi levels[19] E_F are found within this band gap. The Fermi level position is due to the charge distribution, as shown in figure 1.12a.

---

[17] For instance, the laser facility Hercules at the Center for Ultrafast Optical Science (CU-OS) at the University of Michigan provides a laser power of 300 TW at a laser pulse duration of approximately 30 fs. Hercules is thus amongst the most powerful available laser sources.

[18] I.e. the correction of myopia, hyperopia, or astigmatism by re-shaping the cornea via refractive surgery/ cutting of transparent ocular tissue, e.g. for flap preparation.

[19] The Fermi level is the energy level where the occupation probability of charge carriers, e.g. electrons, amounts to 50%.

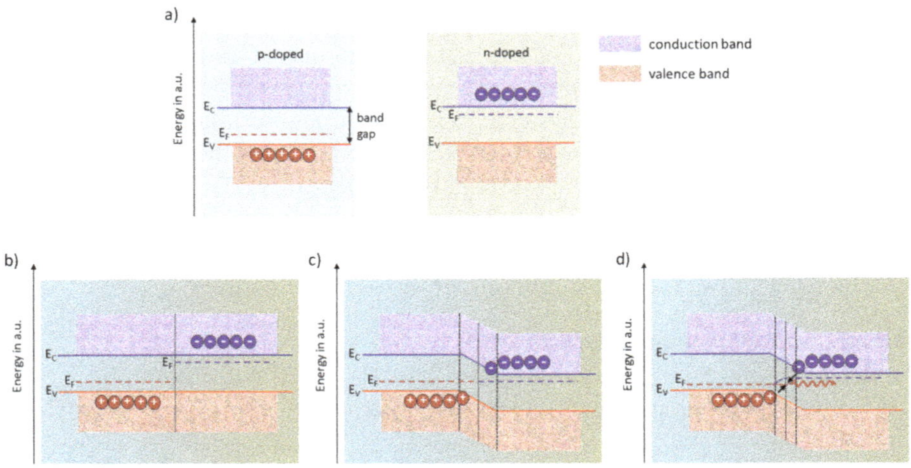

Figure 1.12. Principle of generation of laser light in a diode laser; for detailed description see text.

When contacting both doped semiconductors with different charge distribution and Fermi level position, respectively, as shown in figure 1.12b, this leads to a difference in the position of both involved Fermi levels. However, this state is not possible in thermodynamic equilibrium and the two energy bands, the conduction and valence band with the energy E_C and E_V, respectively, are thus shifted until a common Fermi energy level is formed, as shown in figure 1.12c. As a result the junction becomes free of charge carriers since electrons can diffuse from the n-region into the p-region and positively-charged defects, holes, can diffuse from the p-region to the n-region. When applying a voltage to the semiconductor, the Fermi levels are shifted and the electric-potential barriers are consequently reduced. As shown in figure 1.12d, charge carriers then diffuse into the band gap and electrons and holes recombine. As a result of such recombination, photons are generated by spontaneous emission where the photon energy corresponds to the difference in energy of the energetic states of the involved electrons and holes. Due to the recombination of electrons and holes, photons are then generated by spontaneous emission where the photon energy corresponds to the difference in energy of the energetic states of the involved electrons and holes. When placed in a laser cavity, which is usually given by the polished end surfaces of the semiconductor crystal, as shown in figure 1.13, emission of laser irradiation can be obtained as follows: electrons can exist in the immediate vicinity of holes without any recombination for a certain time, the so-called upper-state lifetime or recombination time. Within this short time of approximately one nanosecond, stimulated emission can be initiated by an incident photon, finally resulting in laser operation by light amplification in the p–n junction zone.

The output power of a single laser diode is limited to approximately 10–40 W. The combination of a number of such single diodes to diode laser stacks allows the realisation of diode laser systems with high output power of up to a number of kilowatts, which allows even industrial materials processing applications. In comparison to other laser types such as solid state lasers or gas lasers, diode lasers

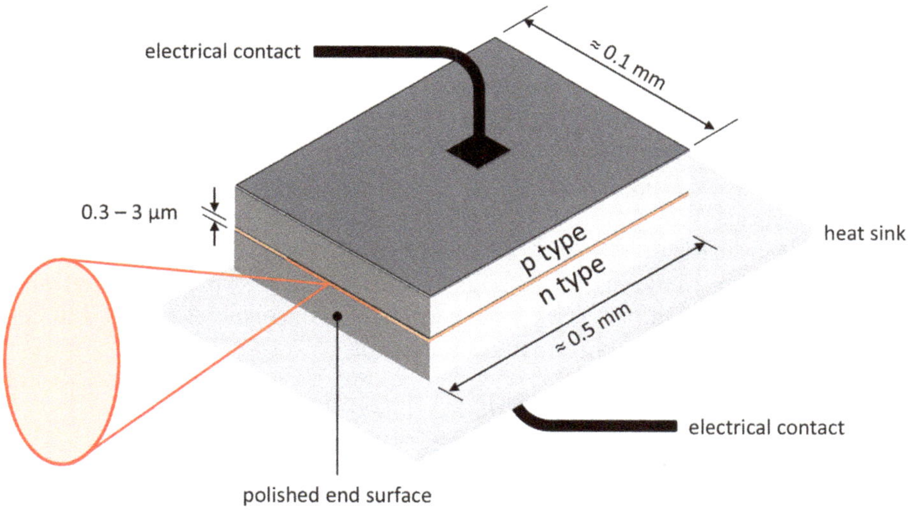

Figure 1.13. Basic setup of a diode laser (adapted from [38]).

Table 1.1. Selection of semiconductor materials used for diode lasers.

Semiconductor material	Formula
Indium gallium phosphide	$In_{1-x}Ga_xP$
Gallium arsenide phosphide	$GaAs_{1-x}P_x$
Aluminium gallium arsenide	$Al_xGa_{1-x}As$
Indium gallium arsenide	$In_xGa_{1-x}As$
Lead cadmium selenide	$Pb_{1-x}Cd_xS$
Lead germanium selenide	$Pb_{1-x}Ge_xS$
Lead germanium telluride	$Pb_{1-x}Ge_xTe$
Indium arsenide antimonide	$InAs_{1-x}Sb_x$
Lead sulfide selenide	$PbS_{1-x}Se_x$
Lead tin selenide	$Pb_{1-x}Sn_xSe$
Lead tin telluride	$Pb_{1-x}Sn_xTe$

feature a number of advantages such as for example a higher degree of efficiency and the possibility to tune the emission wavelength by adjusting the temperature of the semiconductor material[20]. Moreover, diode lasers are very compact and feature a high duration of life. A selection of semiconductor materials used for diode lasers is listed in table 1.1.

[20] The laser wavelength of diode lasers is strongly temperature-dependent due to the temperature-dependence of the band gap energy within semiconductors as described by the so-called Varshni equation. With respect to normal conditions, the laser wavelength is shifted by a 0.3 nm K^{-1} temperature change.

In medicine, diode lasers are either used directly as an actively operating tool in diagnostics and therapy or indirectly as targeting laser or pilot laser for the positioning or adjusting of medical equipment. In diagnostics, diode lasers with low output power are employed as light source for the examination of biological tissue, e.g. for the determination of moving particles such as erythrocytes, i.e. red blood cells, via laser Doppler velocimetry (LDV). The variety of wavelengths of diode laser sources, see figure 1.14, and the accompanying variety of depth of penetration of laser irradiation into tissue further opens a wide range of therapeutic applications. For instance, tissue reactions such as hyperthermia, coagulation, and vaporisation can be obtained. Moreover, diode lasers are suitable light sources for ophthalmic applications or photodynamic therapy.

Properties, parameters and characteristics

- Laser active gain medium: doped semiconductors.
- Emission wavelengths: typically 350 nm to 11 μm, but up to 50 μm possible.
- Extremely high duration of life (theoretically up to 100 years).
- Compact and light setup.

Applications in medicine

- Light source in diagnostics, e.g. for detection of blood flow velocity via laser Doppler velocimetry (LDV) [39, 40].
- Realisation of tissue reactions such as coagulation, cutting, vaporisation [41–43].
- Light source for photodynamic therapy (PDT) [44].
- Targeting or pilot laser for medical equipment.

1.2.2 Gas lasers

Ion lasers

In ion lasers, the laser active gain medium is given by ionised inert gases. There are two relevant and well-established ion lasers, the argon-ion (Ar^+) laser and the

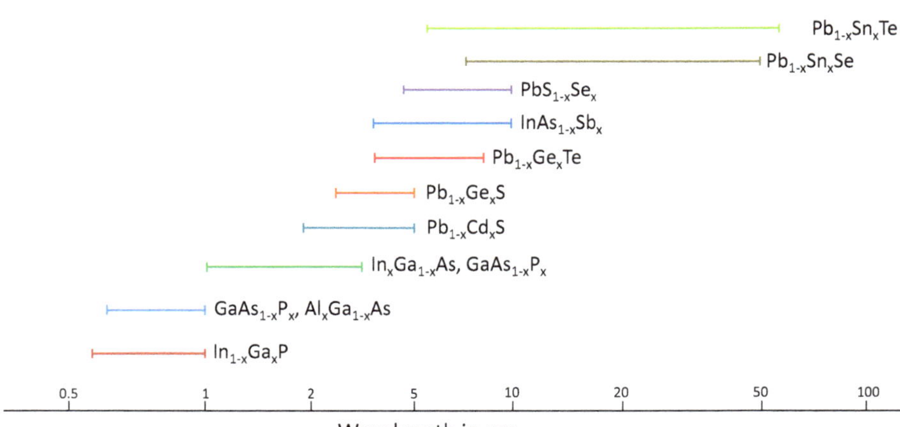

Figure 1.14. Overview of commercially available diode lasers on the basis of the laser active semiconductor material as listed in table 1.1 and the emission wavelength.

krypton-ion (Kr^+) laser. As shown in figure 1.15, the basic setup of such lasers consists of a water-cooled arc discharge tube with an inner diameter of approximately 3 mm, filled with the particular gas at a pressure of about 0.5 mbar. This gas-filled tube thus represents the laser active medium which is placed between the two mirrors of the actual laser resonator.

The tube is made of a material with high thermal conductivity and resistance such as quartz, graphite, or beryllia. The plasma ignited within the tube is confined and compressed towards the tube centre axis by a magnetic field in order to reduce the impact of ion bombardment at the tube wall. In doing so, the efficiency of the actual laser process is additionally increased. Figure 1.16 shows the scheme of an argon-ion laser. Here, argon ions are generated via electron collisions in an electric discharge. As a result of further collisions with electrons, the ions are then excited to different higher energy levels. Emission of laser irradiation finally occurs during the transition from these higher levels to the $4s^2p$ states of argon. It turns out that due to the number of possible excited states and $4s^2p$ states, laser light of several discrete wavelengths in the range from 350 to 530 nm can be generated where the most intense laser lines are found in the visible wavelength range at a wavelength of 488 nm and 514.5 nm, respectively. Moreover, ultraviolet laser irradiation (i.e. at a wavelength of 351 nm and 363 nm, respectively) can be emitted by double ionised argon atoms. The selection of the particularly required or desired laser wavelength can finally be accomplished by introducing an etalon[21] or a dispersive element such as a prism to the ion laser resonator.

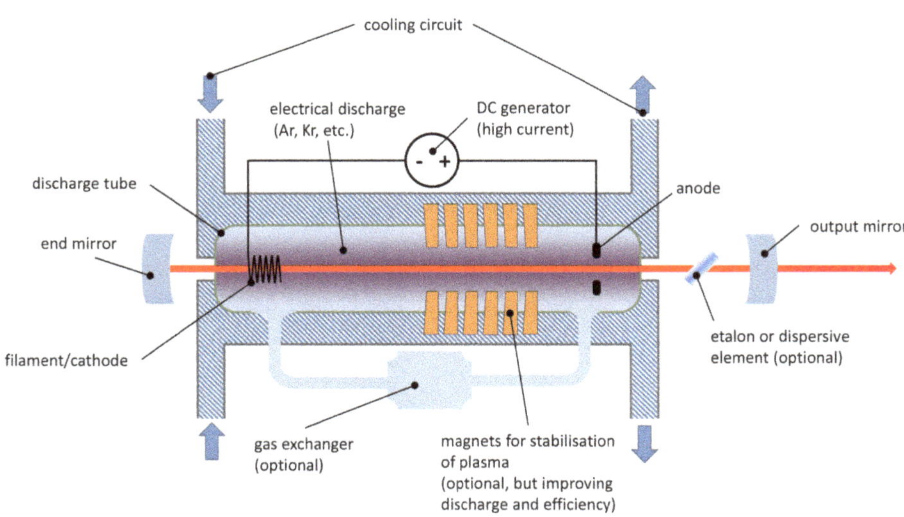

Figure 1.15. Basic setup of an ion laser.

[21] An etalon is a transparent plate with a defined thickness and index of refraction which is placed within the actual laser resonator. There, it acts as second resonator which selectively amplifies the desired longitudinal laser mode and wavelength, respectively, depending on the etalon's thickness and index of refraction, while other modes are suppressed.

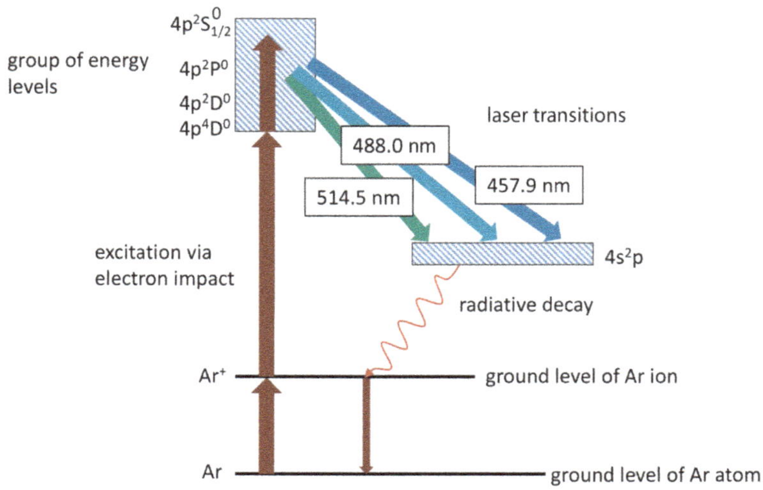

Figure 1.16. Scheme of an argon-ion laser. Ionisation of argon atoms results from collisions with electrons and further collisions leads to an excitation of previously generated argon ions. Laser irradiation is then emitted during the transition from such excited states to the $4s^2p$ states.

Krypton-ion lasers are based on the same working principle as described above. In this case, laser irradiation in a spectral range from 350 to 800 nm is generated. The most intense laser lines are found at 530.9 nm and 568.2 nm, i.e. green laser light, and at 676.4 nm, which is red laser light.

Properties, parameters and characteristics

- Laser active gain medium: ions of inert gases, e.g. argon or krypton.
- Emission wavelengths: 350–800 nm, depending on the inert gas used.
- Efficiency factor: < 1%.
- Pulsed or continuous wave (cw) operation possible.
- Typical pulse duration in pulsed operation: a number of picoseconds.
- Guidance by fibres possible.
- Water cooling necessary.
- Output power up to 30 W (argon-ion laser) and 10 W (krypton-ion laser), respectively.

Applications in medicine

- Treatment of vascular diseases[22] [45–47].
- Removal of pigments [48].
- Laser-based diagnostics, e.g. multi fluorescence microscopy or flow cytometry [49].

[22] Ion lasers are highly suitable for the treatment of vascular diseases since the maximum absorption of haemoglobin is found at approximately 400 nm.

The carbon dioxide laser

The carbon dioxide (CO_2) laser is one of the oldest and most important laser sources in a number of different fields of applications and especially in laser surgery. The gas used for this special type of gas laser is a mixture of helium (82%), nitrogen (13.5%), and carbon dioxide (4.5%) which fills an arc discharge tube as shown in figure 1.17. One should note that the gases which contribute to the actual laser process are nitrogen and carbon dioxide, whereas helium is added in order to increase the efficiency factor of the laser process.

For the generation of laser light, nitrogen molecules are excited by an electric discharge within the tube. The energy is then transferred from the excited nitrogen to CO_2 molecules by collisions, resulting in the actual pumping of the gas mixture. Laser emission in the wavelength range from 9 to 11 μm then occurs between two vibrational states of the CO_2 molecule as shown in figure 1.18 where the strongest lines are found at 10.6 μm and 9.6 μm. The first one arises in the case of a symmetric linear vibration of the involved carbon and oxygen atoms. In contrast, laser irradiation at a wavelength of 9.6 μm is formed during the transition from the upper level to a symmetric bending vibration of the CO_2 molecule.

The processes in such CO_2 lasers can be further supported by adding hydrogen to the gas mixture, resulting in a faster and increased excitation of electrons to a higher energy level. Due to the comparatively high degree of efficiency, CO_2 lasers are even available as battery-driven systems nowadays. However, CO_2 laser irradiation is located in the far infrared wavelength range, restricting the possibilities of beam shaping and guidance. For focussing, refractive components such as lenses made of special IR-transparent materials (e.g. gallium arsenide, GaAs or zinc selenide, ZnSe) are in hand. Beam guidance and transportation is usually performed with the aid of mirror-based jointed arms or hollow-core fibres.

Properties, parameters and characteristics

- Laser active gain medium: gaseous carbon dioxide.
- Gas mixture (typical): CO_2:N_2:He – 1:1:8.
- Emission wavelengths: 10.6 μm and 9.6 μm.

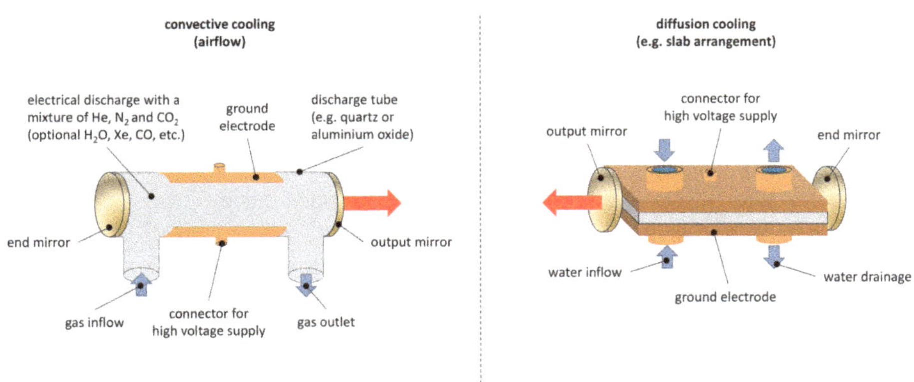

Figure 1.17. Basic setup of a CO_2 laser.

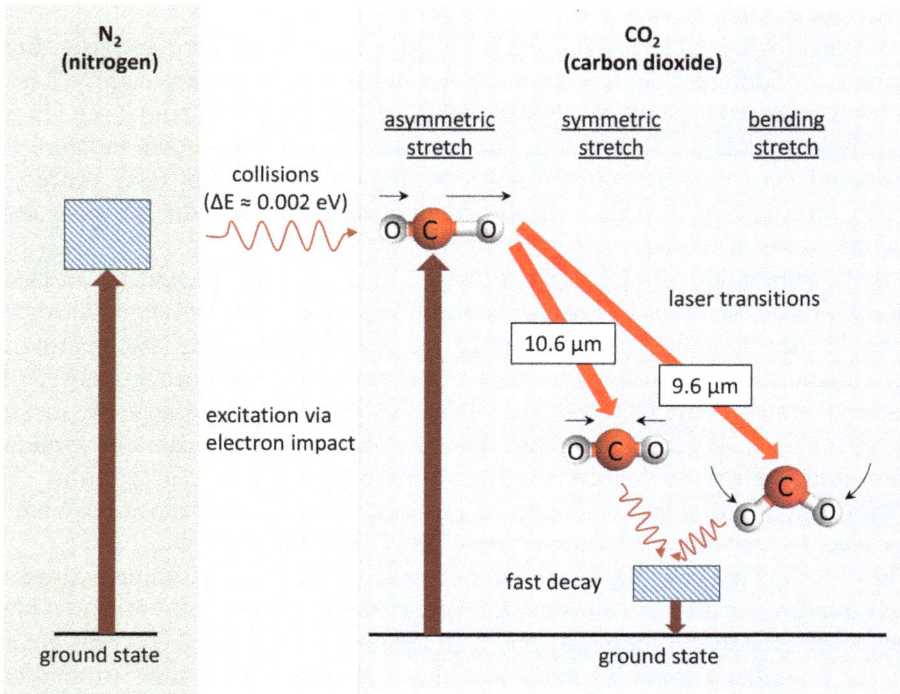

Figure 1.18. Energy levels of a CO_2 laser including the vibrational modes of the CO_2 molecule and the laser transitions at 10.6 μm and 9.6 μm.

- Efficiency factor: up to 30%.
- Pulsed or continuous wave (cw) operation possible.
- Simple and robust setup without any hazardous gases.
- Laser power: up to a number of megawatts in cw operation.
- Beam guidance by mirror systems.
- Penetration depth into tissue: some tens of microns (typically 10–30 μm).

Applications in medicine
- Classical laser for cutting soft and hard tissue as well as bones in surgery [50–52].
- Dermatological applications for the removal of superficial skin alterations such as verrucas.
- Laser-based diagnostics, e.g. monitoring of anaesthesia.
- Special applications, e.g. transmyocardial laser revascularisation (TMLR) in cardiology or partial removal of kidney in urology [53, 54].

The helium neon laser
The helium neon (HeNe) laser was the first continuous wave laser ever and is one of the most important laser sources in modern measurement technology. For laser

operation, the actual laser active gain medium is neon whereas helium is added in order to support the excitation process (comparable to the function of helium in carbon dioxide lasers). A typical gas composition for HeNe lasers is 1 mbar of helium and 0.1 mbar of neon. This gas mixture is filled into an arc discharge tube where a direct current or radio frequency discharge is ignited. The electrons generated in this way cause the excitation of helium atoms to different higher excited states, finally accumulating in the comparatively long-lasting metastable states 2^3S and 2^1S, as shown in figure 1.19.

These metastable states show energies quite similar to two selected states, 2s and 3s, of the neon atom, which can thus be easily excited via two-body collisions, resulting in a resonant energy transfer from excited helium to neon and a population inversion at the above-mentioned higher states of neon. Laser light is finally emitted during the de-excitation from higher s-states to lower p-states[23] of the neon atom. As a result of the number of possible transitions between these states, helium neon lasers can be operated at quite different wavelengths in the visible and infrared spectral ranges up to 3391.3 nm. However, the most commonly used helium neon laser wavelengths are 543.3 nm and 632.8 nm. In medicine, this type of laser is mainly used as a targeting or pilot laser for alignment, but also as a light source for applications in spectroscopy or even for therapeutic purposes like for example bio-stimulation.

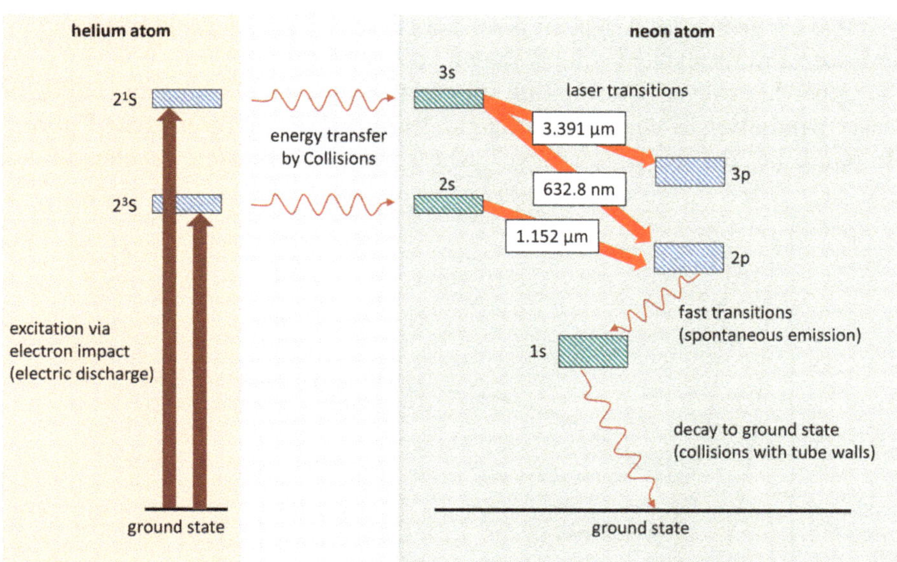

Figure 1.19. Scheme of energy levels of helium and neon including the dominant transitions.

[23] The abbreviations s and p refer to the atomic orbitals.

Properties, parameters and characteristics

- Laser active gain medium: gaseous neon.
- Gas mixture (typical): He:Ne – 10:1.
- Emission wavelengths: 543.3 nm (green), 594.1 nm (yellow), 611.8 nm (orange), 632.8 nm (red), 1152.3 nm (infrared), 1523.1 nm (infrared), and 3391.3 nm (infrared).
- Efficiency factor: < 1%.
- Laser power: typically 1–5 mW, up to 100 mW possible.
- Beam guidance by fibres possible.

Applications in medicine

- Classical targeting or pilot laser.
- Light source for spectroscopy in diagnostic.
- Light source for therapeutic applications.

The excimer laser

The excimer laser is a special type of gas laser which exclusively emits laser irradiation in the ultraviolet wavelength range from 126 to 351 nm. Its laser active gain medium consists of so-called excited dimers, which is the origin of the abbreviation 'excimer'. Suitable dimers are noble gas dimers such as argon (Ar_2) or xenon (Xe_2) or noble gas halide bonds, e.g. argon fluoride (ArF) or xenon chloride (XeCl). In contrast to solid or other gaseous laser gain media, these compounds do not feature a stable ground state, but a stable excited state. A typical potential curve of a noble gas halide bond in the ground state and the excited state is shown in figure 1.20.

The upper laser level is formed by the electrically excited noble gas halide bond and laser irradiation is emitted during the transition to the non-excited noble gas halide bond, i.e. the lower laser level, where the emitted laser wavelength results

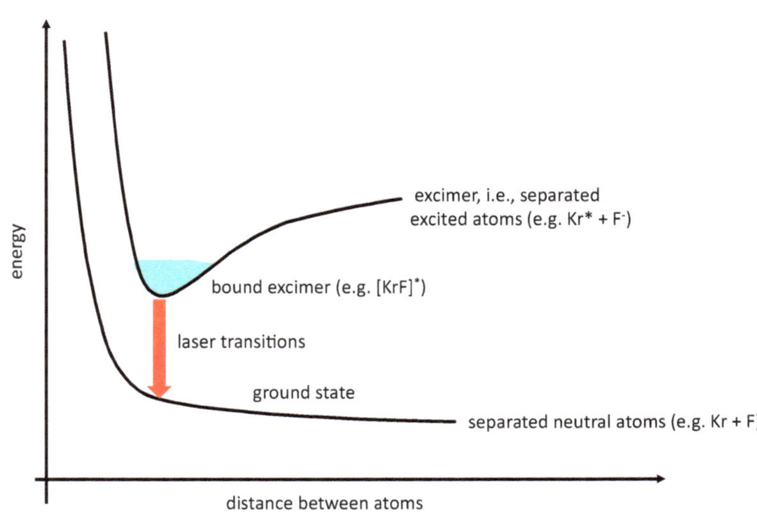

Figure 1.20. Typical potential curve of a noble gas halide bond; '–' denotes negatively charged compounds and '*' denotes the excited state (adapted from [12]).

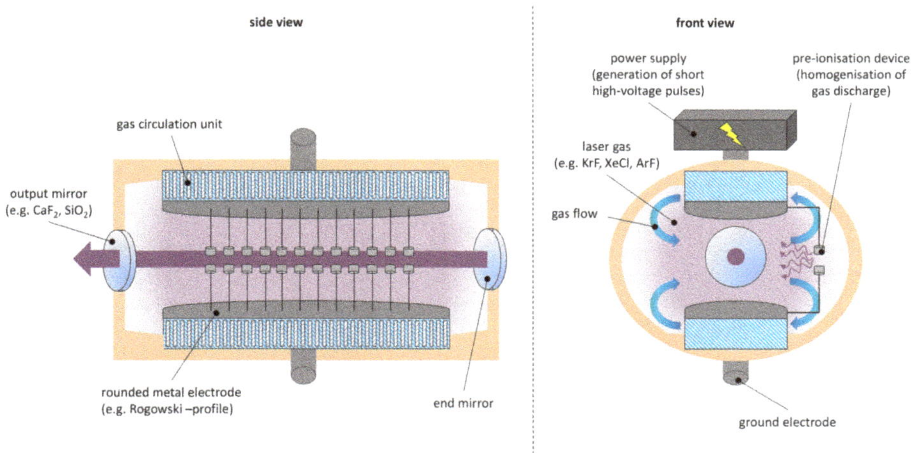

Figure 1.21. Basic setup of an excimer laser (adapted from [12]).

from the potential difference of both levels. The noble gas halide bond is no longer stable after this mechanism has taken place. It thus decomposes into a noble gas atom and a halogen atom within a number of picoseconds after the actual laser process. In order to initiate this process, the gas mixture is brought between two high-voltage electrodes[24], as shown in figure 1.21, and excited by an electric discharge.

This electric discharge can be classified into two stages: first, free electrons are generated between the electrodes by a primary discharge, allowing a homogenous ignition by the subsequent main discharge. As a result of this principle of excitation, excimer lasers can only be operated in the pulsed regime where the pulse duration typically amounts to ten to some hundreds of nanoseconds. Even though buffer gases, for example helium or neon, are further added to the actual laser active gas mixture in order to increase the efficiency of the laser process, the degree of efficiency of excimer lasers is quite low and merely amounts to 2–4%. However, this type of laser allows the generation of discrete laser wavelengths in a broad UV wavelength range including the UV-A, UV-B, and UV-C[25] sub-ranges, as listed in table 1.2.

Properties, parameters and characteristics

- Laser active gain medium: excited dimers.
- Emission wavelengths: 126–351 nm.
- Efficiency factor: 2–4%.
- Laser power: typically 200 W.
- Exclusively pulsed operation possible.
- Water cooling required.
- Partially use of hazardous gases (e.g. fluorine, chlorine).

---

[24] The length of the electrodes can be up to 1 m.

[25] For instance, this wavelength range is highly suitable for disinfection by ultraviolet germicidal irradiation (UVGI).

Table 1.2. Overview of gases and gas mixtures used in excimer lasers including the particular discrete wavelength and the corresponding ultraviolet (UV) wavelength sub-range of emitted laser irradiation.

Gas/gas mixture	Symbol/molecular formula	Laser wavelength in nm	UV range according to ISO 21348
Argon	Ar_2	126	UV-C
Fluorine	F_2	157	UV-C
Xenon	Xe_2	172	UV-C
Argon fluoride	ArF	193	UV-C
Krypton chloride	KrCl	222	UV-C
Krypton fluoride	KrF	248	UV-C
Xenon bromide	XeBr	262	UV-C
Xenon chloride	XeCl	308	UV-B
Xenon fluoride	XeF	351	UV-A

Applications in medicine

- Special applications in neurosurgery, e.g. excimer laser assisted non-occlusive anastomosis (ELANA) [55, 56].
- Laser assisted *in situ* keratomileusis (LASIK) in ophthalmology [57–59].

1.2.3 Dye lasers

Dye lasers could also be referred to as liquid lasers since the laser active medium is a radiant dye[26], dissolved in a carrier liquid[27]. In contrast to most other laser sources, dye lasers can be tuned within a broad range of laser wavelengths. For a single dye, the range amounts to 50–100 nm and the availability of a number of different dyes, see figure 1.22, allows the generation of laser irradiation in the visible and near infrared wavelength range from 400 to 900 nm.

The well-established and widely used dye Rhodamine 6G, for instance, emits laser light in the green and yellow wavelength range from 555 to 585 nm where the maximum is found at 566 nm. In a dye laser setup, shown in figure 1.23, the particular dye is dissolved in a carrier liquid such as methanol and placed in a cuvette. In practice, the liquid is permanently circulated by a pump circuit and cooled in order to exchange and to regenerate the liquid volume which is subject to the pump energy which induces population inversion. Pumping is performed optically by flash lamps or laser irradiation from solid state pump lasers, usually Nd:YAG lasers. In the first case, the cuvette is placed within an elliptical or cylindrical mirror and the light emitted by the flash lamp is focussed into the liquid, resulting in the excitation to a higher laser level and the subsequent generation of laser irradiation.

[26] From a chemical point of view, radiant dyes are aromatic molecules which feature conjugated double bonds.

[27] The discovery of the dye laser was one of the fortunate coincidences in the history of science. In 1966, Fritz P Schäfer performed experiments using a ruby laser. By accident, the laser beam was sent through a cuvette filled with a fluorescent dye. Since the glass walls of the cuvette acted as laser resonator, the ruby laser pumped the dye which therefore emitted its proper and particular laser irradiation.

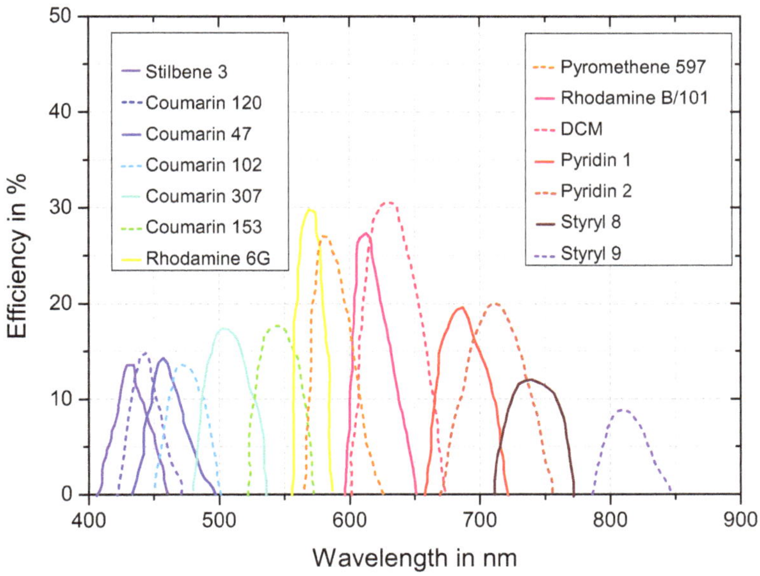

Figure 1.22. Overview of different laser active dyes for generating laser irradiation in the visible and infrared wavelength range (adapted from [12]).

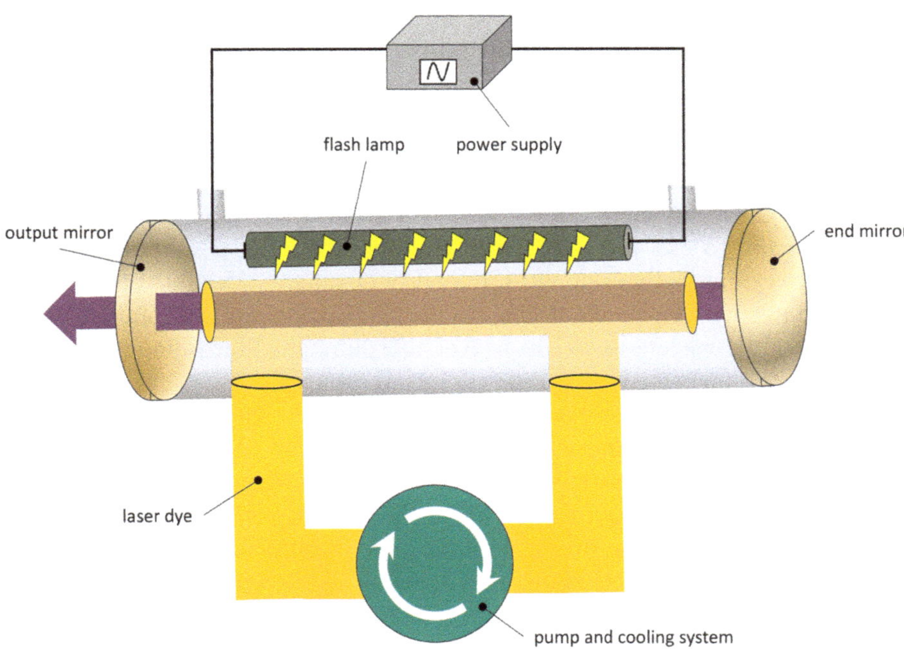

Figure 1.23. Setup of a flash lamp-pumped dye laser (adapted from [12]).

Properties, parameters and characteristics

- Laser active gain medium: fluorescent, radiant dyes.
- Emission wavelengths: 400–900 nm.
- Spectral bandwidth of single dye: 50–100 nm.
- Efficiency factor: approximately 0.5%.
- Pulsed or continuous wave (cw) operation possible.

Applications in medicine

- Treatment of vascular malformation (dysplasia) in dermatology [60, 61].
- Light source for spectroscopy for the examination of tissue[28] [62].
- Light source for laser scanning microscopy (LSM) in diagnostic.

1.3 Laser safety aspects

In industrial use, laser irradiation is capable of cutting and drilling steel and other hard and resistant materials. It is thus obvious that the careful choice of appropriate laser irradiation as well as the knowledge and consideration of laser safety aspects becomes crucial when applying lasers in medicine. If improperly used laser irradiation is a potential direct health risk but also bears secondary hidden risks. Primary, direct risks are laser-induced skin or tissue burns and eye damage. The damage mechanisms strongly depend on the laser power/energy or rather the power/energy density and on the wavelength due to wavelength-dependent absorption characteristics of tissue and humours. In particular, the human eye is highly imperilled due to its particular optical properties and its function as a focussing optical system. Figure 1.24 shows the absorbance of the cornea, the anterior ocular chamber, and the eye lens in the characteristic wavelength range from 280 to 360 nm. Within this range, the cornea's absorption increases significantly with decreasing wavelength, whereas the eye lens shows an inverted behaviour.

As a consequence, incident laser irradiation in the UV-B and UV-C wavelength ranging from 100 to 315 nm may cause photokeratitis, i.e. a sunburn-like actinic conjunctivitis. For higher wavelengths in the UV-A range (315–400 nm), the eye lens features high absorption. Incident UV-A laser irradiation can thus induce cataract. Such opacity of the eye lens as well as irreversible damage of the retina may also arise from laser irradiation in the visible and near infrared wavelength range from 380 nm to 1.4 μm. Finally, infrared laser irradiation or light (up to a wavelength of 1 mm) may induce an increased scattering within the interior ocular chamber, also known as aqueous flare[29], or corneal burn. These severe diseases are normally irreversible and have to be avoided absolutely. Even though the natural protective mechanism, the eyelid closure reflex, would normally limit the exposure time to approximately 0.25 s, the use of protective glasses is mandatory when working with high-power lasers. It should be considered that the eyelid closure reflex is only activated in the case of visible light, but not for invisible light in the ultraviolet and infrared wavelength range.

[28] Here, the penetration depth and the resulting depth of information can be adjusted by the choice of the dye and the laser wavelength, respectively.

[29] In physics, this phenomenon is referred to as the Tyndall effect.

Moreover, laser irradiation typically exceeds the critical values in terms of power or energy. In addition to eye damage, laser irradiation may cause severe skin or tissue burns where the interaction of incident laser irradiation and skin or tissue is also strongly wavelength-dependent. As shown in figure 1.25, far ultraviolet and infrared irradiation in the UV-C and IR-B and IR-C wavelength range is absorbed within the outermost layer of the human skin, the stratum corneum.

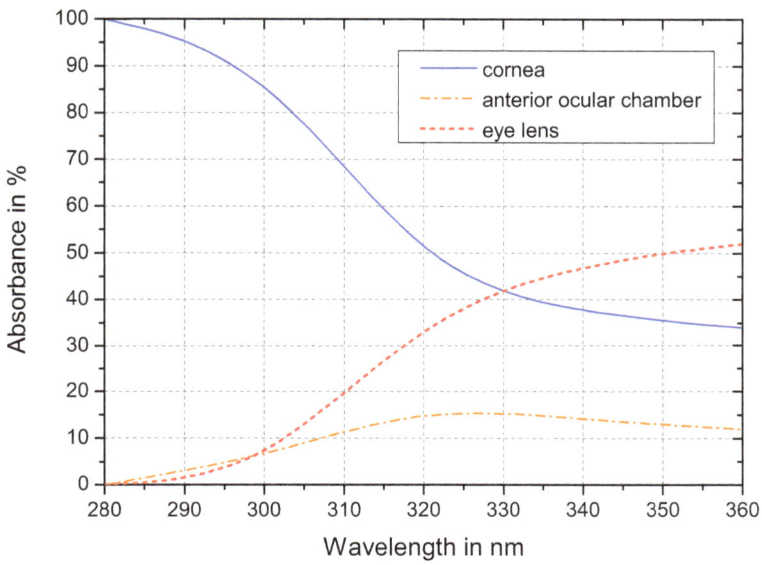

Figure 1.24. Absorbance of the cornea, the anterior ocular chamber and the eye lens versus wavelength in the ultraviolet wavelength range from 280 to 360 nm.

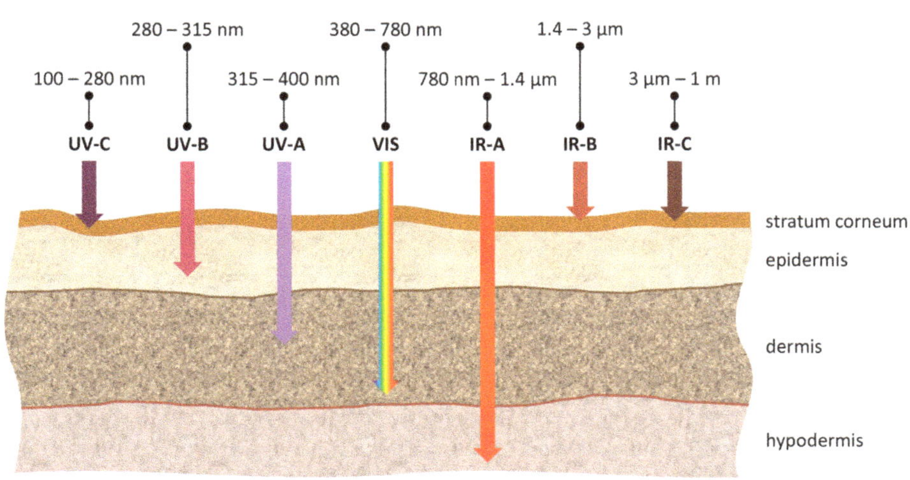

Figure 1.25. Visualisation of the wavelength-dependent depth of penetration of incident light into tissue (adapted from [64]).

UV-B laser irradiation can penetrate into the epidermis, whereas UV-A and visible laser irradiation features a higher penetration depth and can pass through the epidermis with a mean thickness of approximately 100 μm[30] and reach the subjacent connective tissue, the dermis with a thickness in the range from 600 μm to 3 mm. Finally, this dermal layer is even penetrated and crossed by near infrared or IR-A light which thus reaches the subcutaneous tissue, the hypodermis. This wavelength-dependence of the depth of penetration of laser light opens a wide range of different applications in therapy and diagnostics, but also represents a source of danger. In order to avoid skin or tissue burns, protective clothing and gloves should be used. In laser medical applications, the therapist or surgeon, the medical assistants and the patient should wear the appropriate protective clothing and protective glasses.

The aspect of laser safety is covered by different national and international standards. For instance, the requirements for eye protection are specified in the European standard EN 207. EN 208 further regulates the qualification for laser alignment protective glasses. Further aspects of laser safety are finally given in the European standard EN 60825 and the series of standards Z136 of the American National Standards Institute (ANSI Z136). According to these standards, lasers and laser sources are classified into the laser safety classes 1–4[31], as listed in table 1.3. The classification depends on a number of parameters such as the laser wavelength and the maximum permissible exposure (MPE)[32] and accessible exposure limit (AEL), respectively. Further, the beam characteristics in terms of its aperture or focussing are considered.

The aperture of a laser source and the resulting initial beam diameter are also of great interest for the calculation of the nominal ocular hazard distance (NOHD). This parameter takes the divergence of a laser beam into account. In contrast to the idealised description, laser beams do not propagate as a perfectly collimated and parallel beam, but rather feature the shape of a cone over the propagation direction. This widening of the laser beam is quantified by the above-mentioned divergence or divergence angle, usually given in milliradian (abbreviated mrad). The NOHD thus defines the hazard area where direct exposure to laser irradiation can cause eye damage. For continuous wave lasers, it is given by

$$\mathrm{NOHD} = \frac{\sqrt{\dfrac{4 \cdot P}{\pi \cdot \mathrm{MPE}}} - 2w}{\Theta} \tag{1.5}$$

where P is the laser beam power, MPE is the maximum permissible exposure, $2w$ is the initial beam diameter or laser source output aperture, respectively, and Θ is the

[30] Depending on the body region, the thickness of the epidermis varies from approximately 50 μm to 1.4 mm.

[31] Note that according to the old and overridden classification, lasers and laser sources were classified into the laser classes I, II, IIa, IIIa, IIIb, and IV (all class numbers in Roman numerals) and there are notable differences between these old classes and the new ones, 1, 1M, 2, 2M,3R, 3B, and 4 (all class numbers in Arabic numerals).

[32] As an example, the maximum permissible exposure for a single inadvertent exposure of the eye to a continuous wave laser beam with a wavelength between 400 and 700 nm amounts to 25 W cm^{-2}.

Table 1.3. Overview of laser safety classes including the particular wavelength range and maximum accessible exposure limit (AEL) according to EN 60825-1 [63].

Laser safety class	Wavelength	AEL	Note
1	10 nm–1 mm	Cannot be exceeded	Safe under normal conditions, depends on laser aperture
1M	302 nm–4 μm	Cannot be exceeded if not focussed	Safe under normal conditions if not focussed
2	400–700 nm	1 mW (cw, other limits for pulsed lasers)	Safe if eyelid closure reflex limits exposure time to 0.25 s
2M	400–700 nm	1 mW (cw, other limits for pulsed lasers)	Safe if eyelid closure reflex limits exposure time to 0.25 s and if not focussed
3R	302 nm–1 mm	5 mW (cw, other limits for pulsed lasers)	Risks of injury, to be handled carefully
3B	315 nm–1 mm (cw) 400 nm–700 nm (pulsed)	500 mW (cw) 30 mJ (pulsed)	Hazardous if eye is directly exposed
4	10 nm–1 mm	> 500 mW	Most dangerous laser class, bears both direct and indirect risks

divergence angle[33]. Another area of interest is the nominal ocular hazard area (NOHA). It is defined as the area where the laser energy per surface exceeds the maximum permissible exposure on the cornea. Apart from direct health risks such as skin burns and irreversible eye damage, the handling of lasers bears indirect, secondary risks. The mentioned injuries do not exclusively occur as a result of direct exposure to laser light, but also follow from indirect or diffuse irradiation, for example caused by reflecting objects. Jewellery such as rings, bracelets or watches must thus be taken off when working with lasers in general and especially in the case of class 4 lasers. Further, the reflection at surfaces of surgical instruments, clips, forceps, and spreaders should be considered. Finally, another indirect risk is the capability of class 4 laser irradiation of igniting inflammable liquids or media used in medicine such as alcohol-containing germicides, wadding or swabs.

1.4 Laser basics—bottom line

- The term 'LASER' is the acronym for light amplification by stimulated emission of radiation.
- For the generation of laser light, energy is supplied to a laser active medium, leading to the realisation of a population inversion of electrons within the

[33] Note that the NOHD is given in metres; the parameters in equation (1.5) thus have to be inserted in SI or SI-conform units: the laser beam power P is given in watts (W), the maximum permissible exposure MPE is given in watts per square metre (W m^{-2}), the initial beam diameter $2w$ is given in metres (m), and the divergence angle Θ is given in radians.

medium. Emission of laser light then occurs during the subsequent stimulated de-excitation of these electrons.

- The process of supplying energy to the laser active medium is referred to as pumping.
- Amplification of laser light follows from the constructive interference of single light waves generated by stimulated emission.
- As an idealised description, laser light is monochromatic and coherent; it thus features only one colour and wavelength, respectively, and the involved single light waves exhibit no phase delay or retardation.
- The energy of a light or laser photon is given by the product of the frequency of the light wave and Planck's constant.
- For stable laser operation, two laser conditions have to be fulfilled: first, population inversion must be realised initially and second, the amplification of light by constructive interference must be higher than losses of light which occur within a laser resonator.
- Physically, a laser source consists of a resonator which is given by two mirrors, a laser active medium and a pump energy supply for initiating population inversion.
- A basic laser setup delivers continuous wave laser irradiation; pulsed operation is achieved by introducing further active or passive components to the resonator.
- The pulse durations of commercially available laser sources used in medicine vary from the millisecond to the femtosecond range.
- Laser light can be converted into shorter wavelengths by the generation of harmonics of the fundamental laser wavelength employing nonlinear optical effects.
- The wavelengths of available laser sources cover the ultraviolet, visible, near infrared, and infrared wavelength range.
- The classification of laser sources is mainly performed on the basis of the aggregate state of the laser active medium, i.e. solid, gaseous, or liquid (dyes).
- Solid state lasers frequently used in medicine are for example the neodymium–YAG laser, the holmium–YAG laser, the titanium sapphire laser and a number of different diode lasers.
- Gas lasers established in medicine are argon- or krypton-ion lasers, excimer lasers, and carbon dioxide lasers where the latter represents the laser source of highest relevance.
- Dye lasers allow the generation of a comparatively large number of different wavelengths, mainly in the range from 400 to 900 nm.
- The use of laser light bears a number of primary and secondary risks for the therapist, surgeon, medical assistant, and the patient.
- Especially ultraviolet and infrared laser irradiation is well absorbed by the skin and may thus cause severe burns and irreversible tissue damage.
- Lasers are classified into the laser safety classes 1–4 where class 4 represents the most dangerous one.
- Eye protection is one of the most important aspects of laser safety. In order to avoid damage to the eye lens or the retina, appropriate protective glasses

must be worn. In addition, jewellery and watches which may reflect laser light towards the eye must be taken off.

References

[1] White J M, Goodis H E and Rose C L 1991 *Lasers Surg. Med.* **11** 455–61

[2] Launay Y, Mordon S, Cornil A, Brunetaud J and Moschetto Y 1987 *Lasers Surg. Med.* **7** 473–7

[3] Vogel A, Schweiger P, Frieser A, Asiyo M N and Birngruber R 1990 *IEEE J. Quantum Electron.* **26** 2240–60

[4] Lippert B, Teymoortash A, Folz B and Werner J 2003 *Lasers Med. Sci.* **18** 19–24

[5] Fan M, Ascher P, Schröttner O, Ebner F, Germann R and Kleinert R 1992 *J Clin. Laser Med. Surg.* **10** 355–61

[6] Van Hillegersberg R, Van Staveren H, Kort W, Zondervan P and Terpstra O 1994 *Lasers Surg. Med.* **14** 124–38

[7] Albrecht D, Germer C, Roggan A, Isbert C, Ritz J and Buhr H 1998 *Chirurg* **69** 930–7

[8] Marcondes M, Gandolfi Paranhos M P, Spohr A M, Mota E G, Lima da Silva I N, Souto A A and Burnett L H 2009 *J. Biomed. Mater. Res. Part B: Appl. Biomater* **90** 388–95

[9] Liu H C, Lin C P and Lan W H 1997 *J. Endodon.* **23** 691–3

[10] Kilmer S L and Anderson R 1993 *J. Dermatol. Surg. Oncol.* **19** 330–8

[11] Kilmer S L, Lee M S, Grevelink J M, Flotte T J and Anderson R R 1993 *Arch. Dermatol.* **129** 971–8

[12] Berlien H P and Müller G 2000 *Angewandte Lasermedizin—Lehr und Handbuch für Praxis und Klinik* 3rd edn (Berlin: Laser- und Medizin-Technologie) ISBN 3-609-70510-8

[13] Seiler T, Matallana M and Bende T 1990 *J. Refract. Surg.* **6** 335–9

[14] Durrie D S, Schumer D J and Cavanaugh T B 1994 *J. Refract. Surg.* **10** S277–80

[15] Gilling P J, Cass C B, Cresswell M D and Fraundorfer M R 1996 *Urology* **47** 48–51

[16] Gilling P J, Cass C B, Cresswell M D and Fraundorfer M R 1996 *J. Endourol.* **10** 459–61

[17] Erhard M J and Bagley D H 1995 *J. Endourol.* **9** 383–6

[18] Grasso M 1996 *Urology* **48** 199–206

[19] Sofer M, Watterson J D, Wollin T A, Nott L, Razvi H and Denstedt J D 2002 *J. Urol.* **167** 31–4

[20] Walsh J T and Deutsch T F 1989 *Lasers Surg. Med.* **9** 327–37

[21] Walsh J T, Flotte T J and Deutsch T F 1989 *Lasers Surg. Med.* **9** 314–26

[22] Aoki A, Ishikawa I, Yamada T, Otsuki M, Watanabe H, Tagami J, Ando Y and Yamamoto H 1998 *J. Dent. Res.* **77** 1404–14

[23] Hohenleutner U, Hohenleutner S, Bäumler W and Landthaler M 1997 *Lasers Surg. Med.* **20** 242–7

[24] Hibst R and Keller U 1989 *Lasers Surg. Med.* **9** 338–44

[25] Pelagalli J, Gimbel C B, Hansen R T, Swett A and Winn D W 1997 *J. Clin. Laser Med. Surg.* **15** 109–15

[26] Mattioli S, Cremona M, Benaim G and Ferrario A 1991 *Eur. Urol.* **19** 233–5

[27] Alster T S 1995 *J. Am. Acad. Dermatol.* **33** 69–73

[28] Fitzpatrick R E and Goldman M P 1994 *Arch. Dermatol.* **130** 1508–14

[29] Finkel B, Eliezri Y, Waldman A and Slatkine M 1997 *J. Clin. Laser Med. Surg.* **15** 225–9

[30] Nanni C A and Alster T S 1999 *J. Am. Acad. Dermatol.* **41** 165–71

[31] Reid W, McLeod P, Ritchie A and Ferguson-Pell M 1983 *Br. J. Plast. Surg.* **36** 455–9

[32] Leuenberger M L, Mulas M W, Hata T R, Goldman M P, Fitzpatrick R E and Grevelink J M 1999 *Dermatol. Surg.* **25** 10–4

[33] Taylor C R, Gange M and Dover J S 1990 *Arch. Dermatol.* **126** 893–9

[34] Wimmershoff M B, Scherer K, Lorenz S, Landthaler M and Hohenleutner U 2000 *Dermatol. Surg.* **26** 205–10

[35] Bindewald-Wittich A, Han M, Schmitz-Valckenberg S, Snyder S R, Giese G, Bille J F and Holz F G 2006 *Invest. Ophthalmol. Vis. Sci.* **47** 4553–7

[36] Cahalan M D, Parker I, Wei S H and Miller M J 2002 *Nat. Rev. Immunol.* **2** 872

[37] Lubatschowski H, Maatz G, Heisterkamp A, Hetzel U, Drommer W, Welling H and Ertmer W 2000 *Graefeas Arch. Clin. Exp. Ophthalmol* **238** 33–9

[38] Brunner W and Junge K 1989 *Wissensspeicher Lasertechnik* (Leipzig: VEB Fachbuchverlag)

[39] Huang X, Lu L, Gush R and Boggett D 1996 A new, fast, high resolution laser doppler imager for clinical and research use *Proc. 6th World Congress for Microcirculation (Munich, Germany, August 1996)*

[40] De Mul F, Van Spijker J, Van der Plas D, Greve J, Aarnoudse J and Smits T 1984 *Appl. Opt.* **23** 2970–3

[41] Goharkhay K, Moritz A, Wilder-Smith P, Schoop U, Kluger W, Jakolitsch S and Sperr W 1999 *Lasers Surg. Med.* **25** 401–6

[42] Pirnat S 2007 *J. Laser Health Acad.* **4** 1–9

[43] Gangi A, Dietemann J L, Guth S, Vinclair L, Sibilia J, Mortazavi R, Steib J P and Roy C 1998 *Am. J. Neuroradiol.* **19** 1955–8

[44] Brancaleon L and Moseley H 2002 *Lasers Med. Sci.* **17** 173–86

[45] L'Esperance F Jr 1969 *Trans. Am. Acad. Ophthalmol. Otolaryngol. Am. Acad. Ophthalmol. Otolaryngol* **73** 1077

[46] Singerman L J 1982 *Retina* **2** 15–28

[47] Apfelberg D B, Maser M R, Lash H and Rivers J 1981 *JAMA* **245** 2073–5

[48] Apfelberg D B, Maser M R and Lash H 1979 *Br. J. Plast. Surg.* **32** 141–4

[49] Schmid I, Uittenbogaart C H, Keld B and Giorgi J V 1994 *J. Immunol. Methods* **170** 145–57

[50] Walsh J T Jr, Flotte T J, Anderson R R and Deutsch T F 1988 *Lasers Surg. Med.* **8** 108–18

[51] Pecaro B C and Garehime W J 1983 *J. Oral Maxillofac. Surg.* **41** 725–8

[52] Garden J M, O'Banion M K, Shelnitz L S, Pinski K S, Bakus A D, Reichmann M and Sundberg J P 1988 *JAMA* **259** 1199–202

[53] Frazier O, March R J and Horvath K A 1999 *New Engl. J. Med.* **341** 1021–8

[54] Aaberge L, Nordstrand K, Dragsund M, Saatvedt K, Endresen K, Golf S, Geiran O, Abdelnoor M and Forfang K 2000 *J. Am. Coll. Cardiol.* **35** 1170–7

[55] Langer D J and Vajkoczy P 2005 *Skull Base* **15** 191

[56] van Doormaal T P, Zwan A v d, Verweij B H, Langer D J and Tulleken C A 2006 *Oper. Neurosurg.* **59** ONS-328–34

[57] Machat J J 1996 *Excimer Laser Refractive Surgery: Practice and Principles* (Slack Incorporated)

[58] Pallikaris I G and Siganos D S 1994 *J. Refract. Surg.* **10** 498–510

[59] Salz J J, Stevens C A and Group L L H S *et al* 2002 *Ophthalmology* **109** 1647–57

[60] Geronemus R G 1993 *J. Dermatol. Surg. Oncol.* **19** 303–11

[61] Garden J M and Bakus A D 1993 *J. Dermatol. Surg. Oncol.* **19** 321–6

[62] Cothren R, Richards-Kortum R, Sivak M, Fitzmaurice M, Rava R, Boyce G, Doxtader M, Blackman R, Ivanc T and Hayes G *et al* 1990 *Gastrointest. Endosc.* **36** 105–11

[63] Gerhard C 2016 *Tutorium Optik: Ein verständlicher Überblick für Physiker, Ingenieure und Techniker* (Berlin Heidelberg: Springer)
[64] Marwitz H 1990 *Praxis der Holografie: Grundlagen, Standard-und Spezialverfahren* (Renningen: Expert-Verlag)

Chapter 2

Basics of medical laser systems

In this Chapter, the general setup of medical laser systems and peripheral components is presented. Different laser beam guidance systems used in medicine such as optical fibres including the mechanisms and restrictions of laser light transport and reasons for losses of light are introduced. In addition to waveguides, frequently-used optical terminal units and handpieces for monitoring and manipulation during laser-based therapy or surgical interventions are discussed. Against this background, different types of contact tips, endoscopes as well as the basic principle of surgical microscopes are presented.

2.1 General setup of medical laser systems

Medical laser systems normally consist of different optical and peripheral devices and several control units. The basic component is a laser source, as introduced in the previous chapter. For safe handling, this laser source is equipped with a shutter unit and connected to a medical-optical terminal unit via a beam guidance system with at least two optical adaptors, as shown in figure 2.1.

The laser source consists of the actual laser, a power supply which feeds the pump energy supply and—as the case may be—the active switch device for the generation of short laser pulses, and a cooling system. A control panel allows easy handling by means of clearly arranged manual control elements. Where necessary, this control panel is also connected to the particular medical-optical terminal unit. The guidance of light from the laser source to the terminal unit can be realised in different ways where normally, either mirror-based jointed arms or optical waveguides are employed, depending on the laser light's wavelength. Basically, the laser source does not significantly differ from a laser source used for other applications such as materials processing or metrology. However, the beam guidance system and the terminal units need to be well-adapted to, or even tailored for, the particular application in laser medicine. An overview of the used systems and devices is given in the following sections.

doi:10.1088/978-0-7503-1275-2ch2

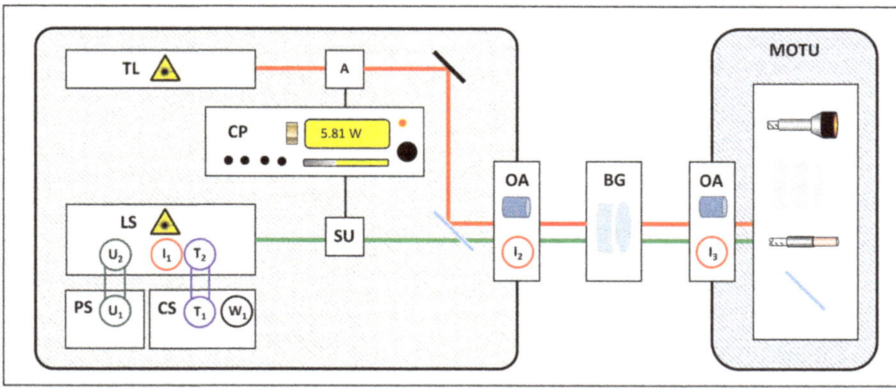

Optical devices
A: attenuator
BG: beam guidance system
LS: laser source
MOTU: medical-optical terminal unit
OA: optical adaptor
SU: shutter unit
TL: targeting laser

Peripheral devices
CP: control panel
CS: cooling system
PS: power supply

Detectors for system monitoring
I: intensity detectors
T: temperature detectors
U: voltage/current sensors
W: water flow detectors

Figure 2.1. Schematic of a medical laser system (adapted from [1]).

2.2 Laser beam guidance systems

As listed in table 2.1, there are three different basic approaches or methods for the guidance of laser beams from the laser source to the particularly used medical-optical terminal unit or device. The direct coupling mentioned there only applies for very compact laser sources and will thus not be discussed in the following sections.

2.2.1 Mirror-based jointed arms

Due to the absorption characteristics of the available optical media the transport of light within bulk waveguides is limited to a certain wavelength range as listed in table 2.1[1]. As a consequence, the transfer of ultraviolet or far infrared light from the laser source to the terminal unit, e.g. a handpiece, a surgical microscope or an endoscope, has to be realised by reflecting instead of refracting optical elements. In practice, this is performed by mirror-based jointed arms. For optimal beam guidance five degrees of freedom are required, three for lateral and axial positioning and two further ones for angular adjustment, as summarised in figure 2.2.

[1] Optical glasses used for the realisation of waveguides are transparent in the wavelength range from approximately 180 nm to 4 μm. For lower or higher wavelengths, optical special materials could be applied, for example calcium fluoride (CaF_2) for the ultraviolet wavelength range or zinc selenide (ZnSe) or gallium arsenide (GaAs) for infrared irradiation such as carbon dioxide laser light. However, mirror-based systems have turned out to be more energy- and cost-efficient and are thus employed in practice.

Table 2.1. Overview of methods for the guidance of laser beams.

Method	Principle	Wavelength range	Advantage	Disadvantage
Direct coupling	Direct propagation of laser beam from output aperture to target through the surrounding air	All wavelengths (except for far ultraviolet range due to absorption of laser irradiation by aerial oxygen)	High beam quality and coherence, polarisation maintaining	Only usable in case of compact laser sources
Mirror-based jointed arms	Guidance of laser beam exclusively by front surface mirrors	All wavelengths, but usually used for ultraviolet and infrared range	High beam quality and coherence, polarisation maintaining	Inflexible and complex setup, sensitive to misalignment
Waveguides	Guidance of laser beams within glassy guides, e.g. by means of total internal reflection	Near ultraviolet, visible, and near infrared range	Flexible, cost-efficient	Restrictions in terms of wavelength, coherence, polarisation and power/energy density

For the user-defined adjustment of a laser beam two tiltable mirrors have to be combined serially. Alternatively, a rotating mirror can be used for this purpose. This approach features a higher achievable precision and is thus established in the production of mirror-based jointed arms for laser beam guidance. Here, the setup as shown in figure 2.2(f), i.e. a serial arrangement of two rotating mirrors with a particular fixed deflection of 90°, is applied since it does not limit the range of possible angles of rotation. Further, mirrors with optimised reflectance can be used due to the fixed angle of incidence of light of 45°.[2] The motion elements of the jointed arms are thus mostly linear stages and pivot bearings. In order to realise one degree of freedom per single motion element, the element must not feature two linear stages or pivot bearings parallel to each other. As a consequence, two sequenced stages or bearings are separated from one another by a deflection unit, normally a cubital joint, leading to a number of possible arrangements and setups of flexibly suspended laser beam guidance systems which feature all the necessary degrees of freedom. Some examples of such systems are shown in figure 2.3. In order to vary the laser beam diameter dynamically, mirror-based jointed arms can contain further

[2] The reflectance of any reflecting surface and especially mirrors is strongly dependent on the angle of incidence (and polarisation) of light as described by the Fresnel equations. Consequently, a mirror coating can be optimised for a certain angle of incidence quite easily, but not for a broad angular range.

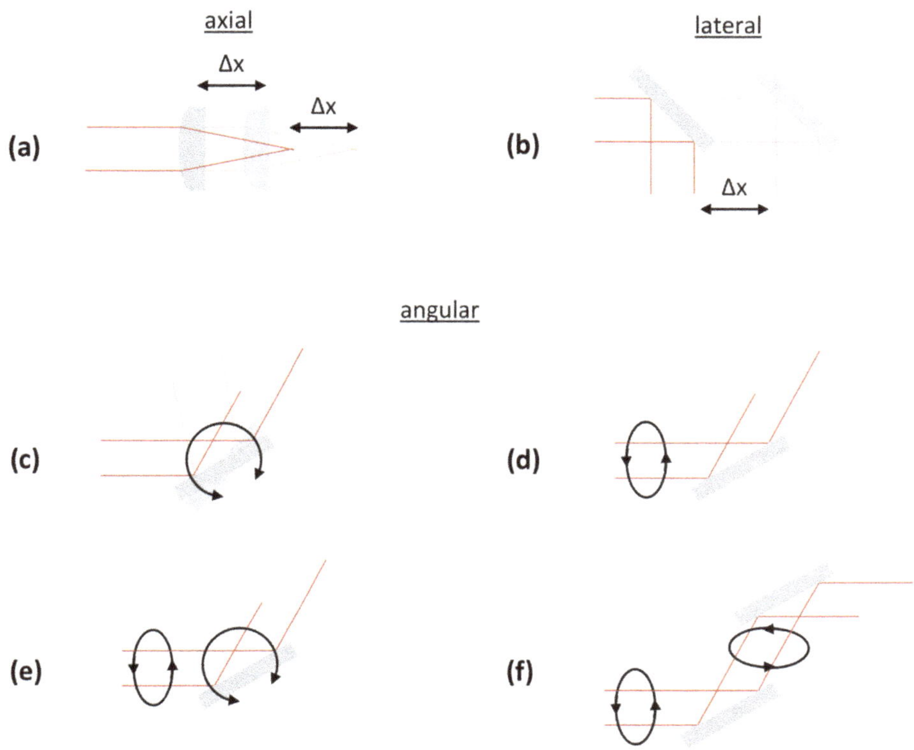

Figure 2.2. Axial, lateral, and angular degrees of freedom for adjusting the position and propagation direction of laser beams (adapted from [1]).

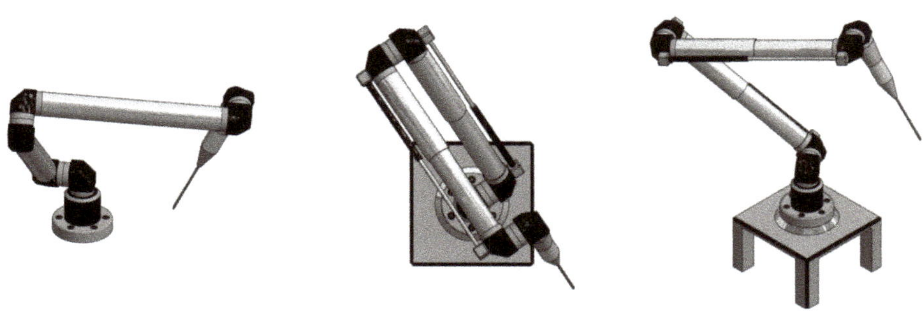

Figure 2.3. Examples of mirror-based jointed arms.

optical elements such as adjustable telescopes[3]. For laser safety reasons, the mirrors and beam path are not bare, but normally housed in tubes.

One has to consider that each element of a jointed arm exhibits a certain mass and misalignment may occur automatically as a result of pure weight, i.e. the force

[3] There are several different approaches for realising a telescope setup. Some are based on lenses (e.g. the Kepler or Galilei type) and some are mirror-based (e.g. the Cassegrain or Newton type). The choice of the particular setup used may thus be decided on the basis of the wavelength of the used laser irradiation.

applied to each element due to gravity. Thus, weight counterbalance becomes necessary. This can be performed by either fixing several counterweights to each hinge of the jointed arm or a total weight fixed on a connecting rod. Such constructs are quite complex and increase the total mass of a jointed arm. In medical use, full weight counterbalance may not be required since the medical-optical terminal units and devices used are operated at some selected, fixed positions. Simpler systems without any counterweights may thus be applied for some medical purposes.

The quality of a jointed arm system is basically characterised by its mass and the angular position accuracy of the laser beam at any position which is realisable by the pivot arm. This parameter is mainly defined by the stiffness of the bearings and hinges and the bending strength of the tubes used. In order to reduce the overall dimension and to allow easy handling, the type of mirror-based jointed arms used has to be adapted to the particular application in medicine if possible.

2.2.2 Optical fibres

Apart from mirror-based systems, optical waveguides can be applied for the transport of light. However, one has to consider the material-dependent restrictions of transmission and the possible laser light wavelength range, respectively, as already mentioned in the previous section. There is a notable number of different waveguides where the optical fibre is the best-known example. This type of waveguide has become established in medical use due to its flexibility and low lateral dimensions[4]. It is applied for both illumination and imaging tasks and represents the core element of any flexible endoscope.

Types of optical fibres

Optical fibres can be classified into three different main categories, hollow core fibres, step index fibres and gradient index (GRIN) fibres. The principles and mechanisms of transportation of light within these optical fibres notably differ and depend on the type of fibre. A hollow core fibre can basically be described as a tube with a reflecting metallic coating applied to the inner tube walls. This type allows the guidance of ultraviolet or far infrared irradiation as for example emitted by carbon dioxide lasers[5]. Another type of hollow core fibre is the so-called photonic crystal fibre (PCF). Here, the guidance of light is based on diffraction and interference at two-dimensional periodic micro structures within the fibre[6] where the structure size is in the range of a quarter of the laser wavelength. Moreover, gradient index (GRIN) fibres and step index fibres are in hand. The latter two types are classical

[4] Optical fibres feature outer diameters of a few hundreds of microns to a number of millimetres and can thus be applied for a number of medical applications such as intravenous diagnostics.

[5] For the realisation of reflecting devices such as hollow core fibres for carbon dioxide laser irradiation at a wavelength of 10.6 μm, gold, copper, silicon, and molybdenum are suitable metals.

[6] Depending on the shape and arrangement of micro structures, two different effects can occur within photonic crystal fibres: first, such a fibre can exhibit a step in the index of refraction and thus work as a classical step index fibre and second, light may be guided due to a photonic band gap.

fibres used in optical communications and transport of light. Step index fibres can further be assigned to two subcategories, multi-mode or mono-mode fibres. As shown in figure 2.4, the only difference between those two types is the diameter of the fibre core.

The typical core diameter of a multi-mode fibre is found in the range from 50 μm to 1.5 mm. As a result, different modes of light can propagate within such a fibre. Simply speaking, these modes are several zigzagged light paths, as shown in figure 2.4(top). Each light path exhibits its proper optical path length[7] and transit time, respectively. This leads to a variation in transit time between all possible modes which are transmitted by such a fibre, known as mode dispersion[8]. This effect can be avoided by reducing the fibre core diameter down to approximately 3–9 μm, depending on the wavelength (and also intensity) of the guided light. As a result, just

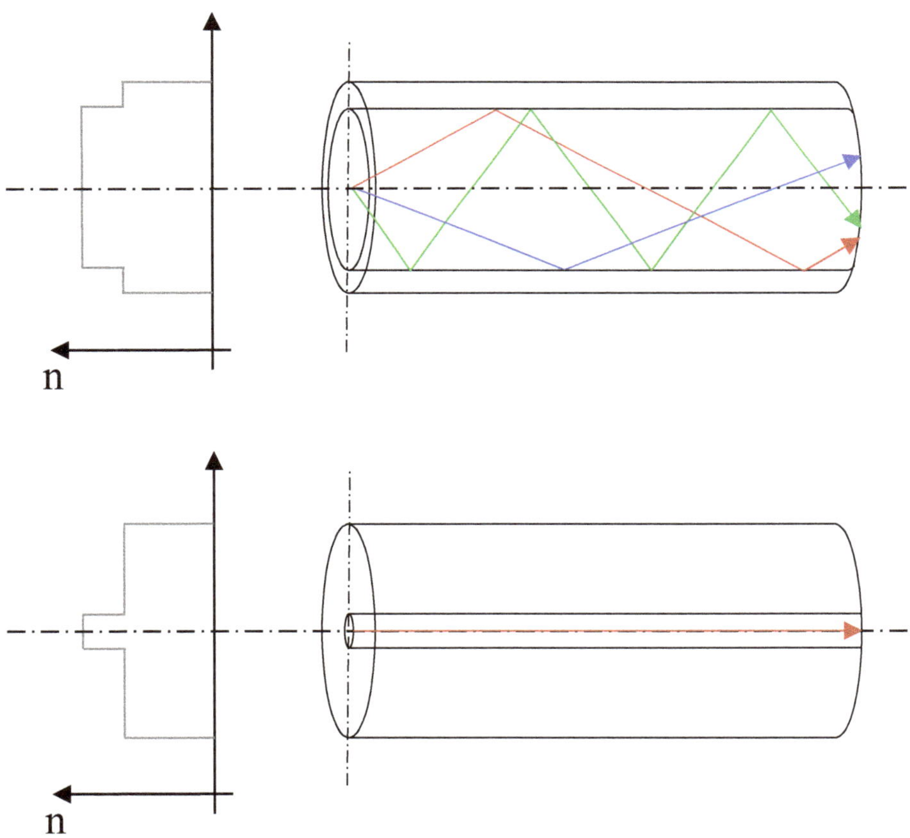

Figure 2.4. The two different types of step index fibres, multi-mode fibre (top) and mono-mode fibre (bottom) including the particular distribution of index of refraction (left) and light guidance (right) (adapted from [2]).

[7] The optical path length is defined as the product of the geometrical length and the index of refraction.

[8] Mode dispersion within multi-mode fibres is not exclusive due to different transit times; it is further amplified by dispersion and scattering mechanisms.

one mode or light wave can propagate within such a fibre (see figure 2.4(bottom)) which is the eponymous functional principle of mono-mode fibres.

Mono-mode fibres used in optical telecommunications may exhibit additional optical functionalities and allow the polarisation of non-polarised light or the maintenance of the initial polarisation state of polarised light. Even though such fibres are currently not used in medical applications, the above-mentioned possibilities may be of interest for future techniques and especially for imaging diagnostics and the development of optical fibre sensors without any electrical device.

A completely different type of optical fibre is the so-called GRIN fibre, where the index of refraction of the core material decreases with increasing distance from the fibre centre[9], as shown in figure 2.5(left).

This decrease, i.e. the distribution of the refractive index n over the radius r of a GRIN lens $n(r)$ is described by a hyperbolic secant distribution (sech), given by

$$n(r) = n_{\text{centre}} \cdot \text{sech}(g \cdot r) \tag{2.1}$$

Here, n_{centre} is the index of refraction at the centre of the GRIN lens and g is its geometrical gradient constant[10]. The guidance of light within such a fibre is due to its radial distribution since incoming light is subject to a continuously altering index of refraction. As a result, mode dispersion is minimised due to the fact that the optical

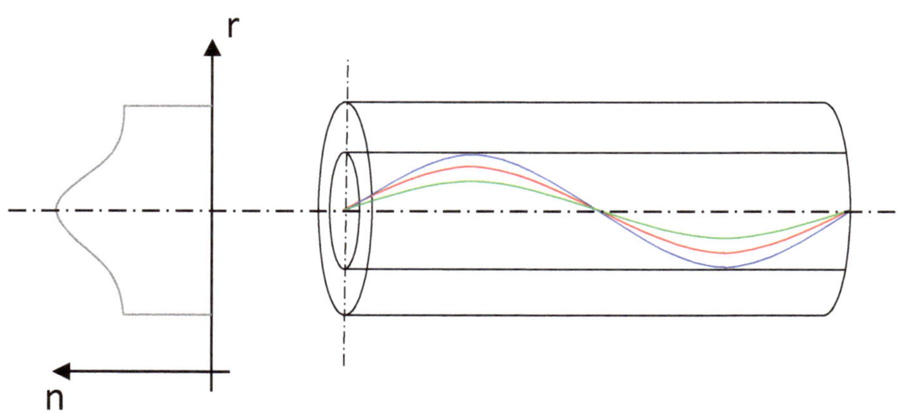

Figure 2.5. Distribution of index of refraction (left) and light guidance within a GRIN fibre (adapted from [2]).

[9] Such a well-defined decrease in index of refraction is achieved by the so-called ion exchange technique where the glass composition is gradually modified. Here, the fibre is dipped into a salt bath and ions are removed from the glass and replaced by ions from the salt bath solution by means of diffusion processes. Since an optical medium's index of refraction is directly related to its composition, this results in a gradual change in its optical characteristic.

[10] In GRIN fibres the geometrical gradient constant is a positive value. However, negative geometrical gradient constants can also be realised. This allows the generation of diverging micro lenses which could be used in micro optical imaging systems at an endoscope's imaging fibre end face for diagnostics.

path length is constant for each possible optical path[11]. The working principle of GRIN fibres thus differs significantly from the mechanism for the transport of light in step index fibres as described in more detail in the following section.

Transport of light in step index fibres

The step index fibre, also referred to as dielectric waveguide, is the most important and widely used type of optical fibre. It basically consists of a core and a cladding made of dielectric media, normally glasses (or plastics in some cases). The light is guided within the core by means of the optical effect of total internal transmission as follows: at an interface from an optically dense medium with the index of refraction n_1 to an optically thinner medium with the index of refraction n_2, light is totally reflected when the angle of incidence corresponds to or exceeds the so-called critical angle of total internal reflection α_{tot}, given by

$$\alpha_{tot} = \arcsin\frac{n_2}{n_1}. \tag{2.2}$$

In an optical step index fibre, such an interface is given by the contact area of the fibre core medium and the fibre cladding where the core medium exhibits a higher index of refraction than the cladding material, $n_{core} > n_{cladding}$, as shown in figure 2.6.

As an idealised description, light is completely reflected at such an interface; total internal reflection is thus virtually free of losses. However, due to a certain overshooting of light into the material with the lower index of refraction[12], the cladding has to feature a certain minimum thickness of approximately 10–20 times the wavelength of the guided light.

As a consequence of its working principle, an optical step index fibre features a critical entrance angle of light α_{max}, see figure 2.6. This angle is the fibre's aperture angle and gives the acceptable angular range or—in a manner of speaking—the field of view of the fibre. Light which hits the fibre entrance surface at higher angles of

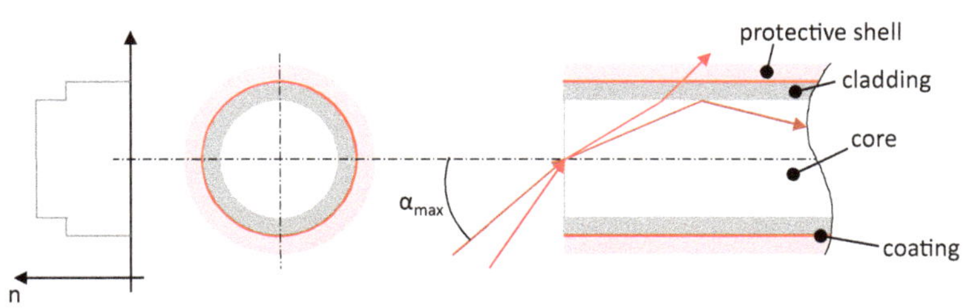

Figure 2.6. Transport of light by total internal reflection within an optical step index fibre (adapted from [1]).

[11] Within GRIN fibres, an optical path with a short geometrical length passes through a zone of higher index of refraction, whereas an optical path with a long geometrical length crosses the boundary area of the fibre where a lower index of refraction is found. On average, both paths thus feature almost the same optical path length.

[12] The depth of penetration of light into the optically thinner medium during total internal reflection amounts to a number of wavelengths of the guided light. This depth range is referred to as the evanescent field.

incidence is consequently not guided by total internal reflection, but enters the cladding according to Snell's law[13], resulting in high attenuation. This effect may even lead to damage of the fibre if laser light is inaccurately coupled into the fibre. Taking equation (2.2) into account, the critical entrance angle of light can be determined according to

$$\alpha_{\max} = \arcsin\left(\sqrt{n_{\text{core}}^2 - n_{\text{cladding}}^2}\right). \tag{2.3}$$

When considering the index of refraction of the ambient medium n_a this essential parameter finally gives a step index fibre's numerical aperture NA,

$$\text{NA} = n_a \cdot \sin\alpha_{\max}. \tag{2.4}$$

If the ambient medium is air with $n_{\text{air}} \approx 1$, the numerical aperture is always smaller than one but increases with increasing index of refraction of the ambient medium according to equation (2.4). This behaviour is used in order to realise large fields of view in microscopy. As shown in figure 2.7, this is achieved by filling the gap between the microscope lens and the sample with a so-called immersion liquid[14]. A selection of such liquids is listed in table 2.2.

Internal damping of optical fibres

In an optical fibre, a certain loss of light over the fibre length occurs due to different mechanisms. This loss is referred to as damping D of the fibre and is usually expressed logarithmically since the reduction in power of light travelling through a fibre is described by an exponential decay. The damping is given by

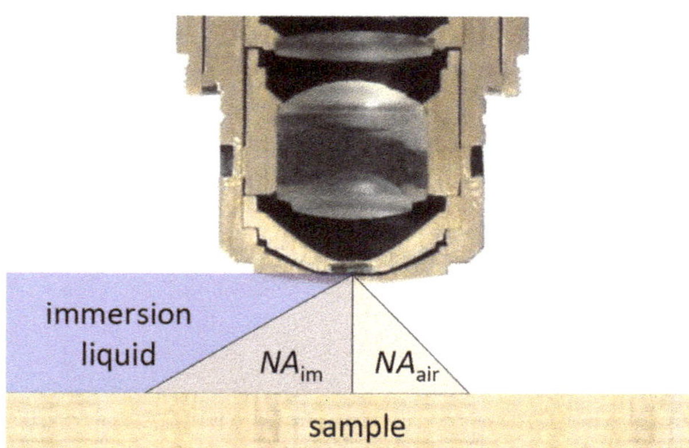

Figure 2.7. Quantitative visualisation of the numerical aperture of a microscope lens with an immersion medium with $n > 1$ (NA_{im}, left) or air (NA_{air}, right) as surrounding medium.

[13] Snell's law quantifies refraction at an optical interface based on the indices of refraction of the involved optical media and the angle of incidence of light. It could be referred to as the most basic law in geometrical optics.

[14] The use of immersion liquids allows the realisation of microscopy setups with an extremely high full field of view of up to 140°.

Table 2.2. Selection of immersion liquids commonly used in microscopy including the particular index of refraction and resulting numerical aperture (in relation to a reference NA of 0.71 in air).

Immersion liquid	Index of refraction n	Numerical aperture NA in relation to NA = 0.71 in air as ambient medium
Water	1.33	0.94
Glycerine	1.47	1.04
Oil	1.52	1.07

$$D = 10 \cdot \frac{1}{l} \log \frac{P_{\text{in}}}{P(l)} \tag{2.5}$$

with P_{in} being the initial power of light coupled into the fibre entrance face. $P(l)$ is the power of light at any position or length l within the optical fibre. Damping is thus a parameter which is directly related to the fibre length; its unit is decibel per length, dB l^{-1}.[15] Damping has several causes such as:

- the absorbance of the core material[16]
- additional absorption and scattering due to material impurities such as inclusions, bubbles[17] and fissures
- geometric-mechanical deviations of the fibre core over its length
- fibre bending, and
- mechanical tension[18].

Moreover, a certain portion of light is lost due to reflection at the fibre end faces. For a single non-coated fused silica surface, the reflectance amounts to approximately 3.5% according to the Fresnel equations. However, this value can easily be reduced to 0.1% or even lower values by applying suitable coatings to the end faces.

The internal damping of fused silica, a well-established optical medium for the core of step index fibres, in the visible wavelength range is mainly due to Rayleigh scattering. This mechanism depends on the glass structure[19] and on wavelength. It decreases with the fourth power of the wavelength. In contrast, damping in the near infrared wavelength range strongly increases with wavelength due to vibrational and rotational absorption bands. As a result, the usable spectral range of transmission of fused silica fibres is limited, as visualised in figure 2.8.

[15] In fibres used for optical telecommunication the base length is usually 1 km. Damping is then given in dB km^{-1}. For fibres with high damping as for example fibres made of special optical materials for the guidance of carbon dioxide laser irradiation, the unit dB m^{-1} is commonly used.

[16] For instance, the absorption coefficient of fused silica amounts to 10^{-5} per cm at a wavelength of 1 μm. According to the Beer–Lambert law, approximately 10% of the incident light is absorbed within this material after a distance or fibre length of 1 km.

[17] Bubbles can easily be formed in the course of the glass manufacturing process and could be described as micro ball lenses made of air or gas within the glass bulk material, giving rise to deflection and scattering.

[18] Mechanical tension in glasses gives rise to birefringence and, in consequence, further losses of light.

[19] The structure of fused silica is given by tetrahedrons consisting of one silicon atom and four oxygen atoms.

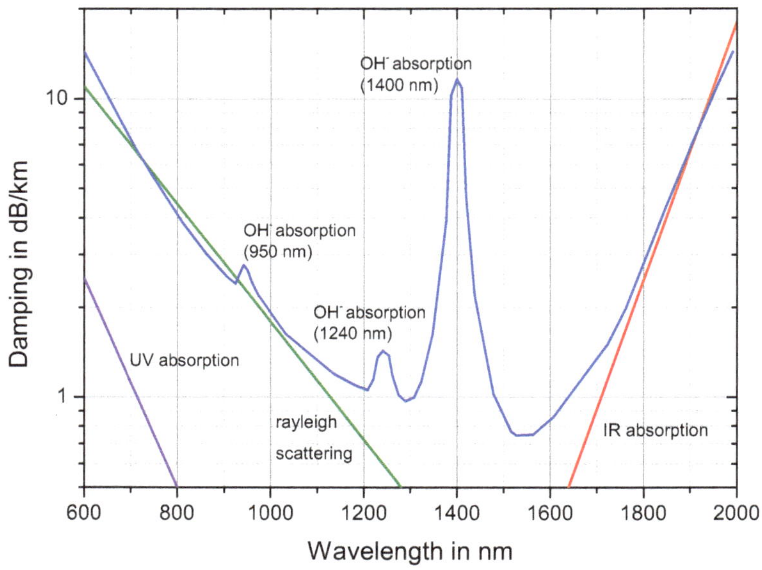

Figure 2.8. Attenuation curve of an optical fibre made of fused silica (logarithmic plotting) (adapted from [2]).

Here, the logarithmic scale allows the easy identification of the above-mentioned influences in the visible and near infrared region. However, even the range of lowest absorption features discrete damping peaks, e.g. at a wavelength of 1400 nm, which are caused by hydroxyl groups within the glass bulk material. Moreover, damping minima, the so-called 'telecommunication wavelengths' at 850 nm, 1.3 μm, and 1.55 μm can clearly be seen.

Bending losses in optical fibres

The numerical aperture not only determines the efficiency of coupling light from diffuse light sources, but also impacts the attenuation of light in bent fibres due to so-called bending losses [3–5]. These types of losses occur due to the fact that the condition of total internal reflection is not valid at the interface from the fibre core to the cladding since the angle of incidence falls below the critical angle of total internal reflection in the bent region of a fibre. In optical telecommunications, where fibres are usually installed without bending or—where necessary—with bending at a high radius, such losses are of the order of 1–2 dB km^{-1}. Since the length of fibres used in medical applications is much shorter, i.e. typically 1 m, these types of losses seem to be irrelevant at first glance. However, bending losses can reach high values in the case of low bending radii R according to

$$N_g = N_0 \cdot \left(1 - \frac{D_{\text{core}} \cdot n_{\text{cladding}}^2}{R \cdot \text{NA}_0^2}\right). \tag{2.6}$$

Here, N_g is the number of modes guided within the bent fibre, N_0 is the number of modes guided in the fibre without any bending, D_{core} is the fibre core diameter,

n_{cladding} is the index of refraction of the cladding material, and NA_0 is the numerical aperture of the fibre without any bending. It turns out that the bending radius not only affects the losses within the fibre, but also its numerical aperture NA (see equation (2.4)). Bent fibres thus feature an effective numerical aperture NA_{eff} which depends on the bending radius R and which is always lower than the NA of the fibre without bending. It is given by

$$NA_{\text{eff}} = \sqrt{n_{\text{core}}^2 - n_{\text{cladding}}^2 \cdot \left(1 + \frac{D_{\text{core}}}{2 \cdot R}\right)^2}. \tag{2.7}$$

This behaviour gains importance in medical applications where low local bending radii occur. For instance, a bending radius of approximately 20 mm is required for entering the coronary artery during cardiovascular laser angioplasty (CVLA). For such low radii as typically needed in medical applications, notable loss in transmitted laser power may occur, as shown in figure 2.9. It can finally be summarised that fibres with high numerical apertures and thick cores are less prone to bending losses [6].

Figure 2.9 visualises the well-known expression for the bending losses:

$$B_1 \propto \frac{n^2}{NA^2} \cdot \frac{D_{\text{core}}}{r_b} \tag{2.8}$$

where B_1 is the bending losses and r_b the bending radius, respectively. In medical applications, bending losses not only reduce the efficiency of transport of light by step index fibres, but bear several secondary risks. First, laser light leaving the fibre at bent zones may jeopardise the therapist, surgeon, medical assistant and the patient. Second, the fibre could be destroyed locally and glass splinters could

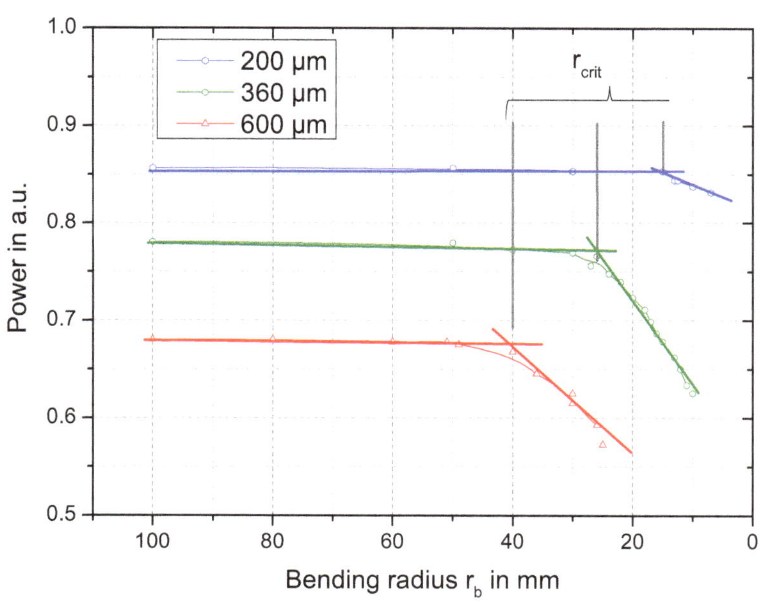

Figure 2.9. Change of power transmission within optical fibres versus bending radius.

consequently enter the vascular system or emergent laser light could burn or even perforate cell and vein walls. Third, the fibre end could be cut off and remain within the vein, making a subsequent invasive surgical intervention necessary.

Power limits of optical fibres

The possibility of transporting light within optical fibres is not only restricted by wavelength, but also by the power or energy of the guided laser irradiation. High power or energy usually results in damage of the fibre which may also occur in the case of laser sources with low output power or energy, but high power or energy density. For instance, high densities occur in GRIN fibres due to the functional principle of this type of fibre and the accompanying continuous focussing and defocussing of light during propagation. A selection of laser-induced damage thresholds (LIDT) of optical fibres is listed in table 2.3.

The data listed here are guidance values. In practice, the LIDT may differ significantly since it depends on a number of different influencing factors, for example:

- the quality of the fibre end face
- the laser pulse duration
- the laser wavelength
- the number of applied laser pulses, and
- the way of focussing.

Influence of the fibre end face quality

Different qualities of a fibre's end faces may result from the particular manufacturing method. Basically, an end face of an optical fibre can be generated in different ways, (i) breaking where the fibre is cleaved by scoring the cladding and subsequent breaking, (ii) fire polishing where the fibre is cut and the end face is then polished by heating the glass and self-organised smoothing due to surface tension of the glass melt, and (iii) classical polishing[20]. Broken fibre end faces feature the highest LIDT and classically polished ones the lowest LIDT.

Table 2.3. Selection of laser-induced damage thresholds LIDT of optical fibres [7–9].

Laser type	Wavelength	Pulse duration	LIDT
Nd:YAG	1064 nm	5–20 ns	0.5–8 GW cm^{-2}
Nd:YAG	1064 nm	100–150 ns	100 MW cm^{-2}
Nd:YAG	1064 nm	Continuous wave	$\approx$5 MW cm^{-2}
Excimer	308 nm, 351 nm	15 ns	$\approx$0.5 GW cm^{-2}
Excimer	308 nm, 351 nm	150–25 ns	100 MW cm^{-2}

[20] Classical polishing, also referred to as chemical–mechanical polishing (CMP), is performed with the aid of polishing agents is aqueous solution. This process usually gives rise to the formation of a hydrated layer on the actual fused silica glass surface of the fibre core due to hydrolytic scission. Such hydrated layers exhibit comparatively high absorption and low laser-induced damage threshold, respectively.

Influence of the laser pulse duration

The pulse duration τ of pulsed laser irradiation is directly related to the damage threshold: when expressed as maximum power density, i.e. the maximum intensity $I_{\max}$, the damage threshold of a fibre surface is in inverse proportion to the square root of the pulse duration according to

$$I_{\max} \propto \frac{1}{\sqrt{\tau}} \tag{2.9}$$

When referring to the energy density, also known as fluence F, the damage threshold is proportional to the square root of the pulse duration,

$$F \propto I_{\max} \cdot \sqrt{\tau} \tag{2.10}$$

which is valid for the pulse duration range from a number of picoseconds to some tens of nanoseconds.

Influence of the laser wavelength

Optical fibres feature some significant absorption maxima, as shown in figure 2.10. The laser wavelength λ is thus an essential parameter which might contribute to fibre damage by means of absorption of light. Moreover, it should be noted that the shorter the laser wavelength, the higher the photon energy according to equation (1.2), leading to a decrease in damage threshold in the ultraviolet wavelength range.

Influence of the number of applied laser pulses

In comparison to single pulses, the application of multiple pulses significantly reduces the laser-induced damage threshold where a reduction by a factor of at least two is reported in the literature. This is due to the fact that the energy of single pulses may accumulate, resulting in an effectively applied amount of laser energy. This is

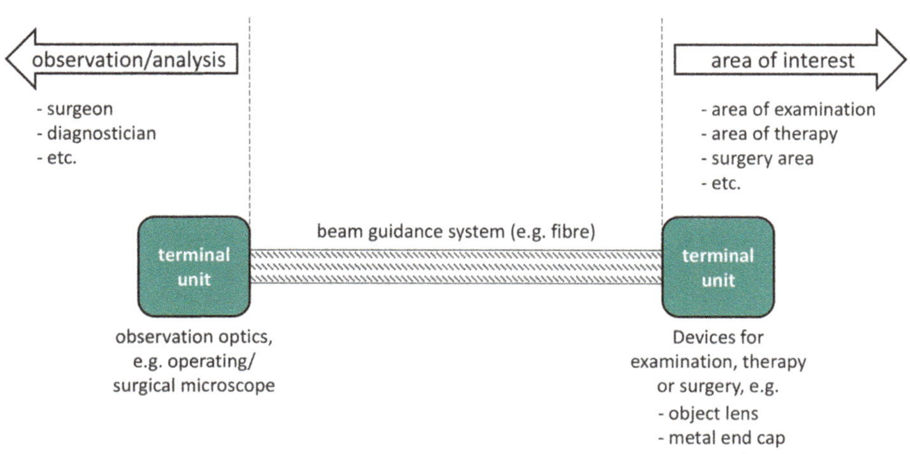

Figure 2.10. Overview of the two spaces connected via beam guidance systems, the observation or analysis area (left) and the area of interest (right) including a selection of frequently used optical terminal units.

usually quantified by the so-called laser dose D[21], i.e. the product of the pulse energy E of the single laser pulses and the number of applied laser pulses N. Moreover, the laser pulse repetition rate, i.e. the number of laser pulses per second, has a notable impact where high repetition rates result in low LIDT due to the accumulation of incident laser energy and the shorter time for thermal relaxation processes.

Influence of the way of focussing
During the focussing of laser light onto a fibre entrance surface the position of the focal point with respect to the optical interface of the surrounding medium and the glass is a critical parameter. It may strongly impact the coupling of light into the fibre and cause damage at the end face or within the fibre bulk material. Generally, the fluence within the focal point should be lower than the damage threshold fluence.

2.3 Optical terminal units and accessories

In practical laser technology, for example medical applications, any laser beam guidance system is equipped with optical terminal units at its entry and exit. The particular type of terminal unit strongly depends on its specific position where two spaces, the observation or analysis area and the area of interest can be identified, as shown in figure 2.10.

In the observation or analysis area, the surgeon or diagnostician uses suitable observation optics such as magnifying lenses or even operating or surgical microscopes in order to monitor surgical interventions or to analyse conspicuous features on tissue surfaces within the area of interest. This area is thus the area of examination, therapy or surgery. Here, suitable terminal units are employed for different purposes. For instance, object lenses allow the intravascular examination at high fields of view and metal end caps or contact tips are used as either therapeutic or surgical instruments. Moreover, light sources for illumination are required. The simplest type of medical-optical terminal units is the blank polished end face of an optical fibre or a catheter with integrated waveguide. Introducing surgical handpieces or contact tips to fibre end faces further allows the realisation of terminal units with quite different functionalities, depending on the particular application. For instance, the use of focussing or defocussing optical elements opens a wide range of possibilities and even endodontic retreatment or intravascular microsurgery, e.g. anastomosis procedures, are made possible by the use of sophisticated optical terminal units or systems such as operating microscopes.

Optical waveguides and the associated optical elements and systems are usually combined with miniaturised electro-optic and mechanical components in endoscopes. Such endoscopic systems are used in diagnostics and minimally invasive surgery to an increasing degree. Here, it has to be differentiated between two main methods of applying medical-optical terminal units, the contact method and the

[21] In this context, the term 'dose' is a specific technical term used in laser technology and should not be confused with the terms 'dose' or 'dose rate' used in medicine.

distance method. In the first case, the terminal unit is brought into direct contact with the tissue to be treated, for example for laser-induced carbonisation, coagulation, or cutting. Working without any direct contact of the terminal unit and the tissue is referred to as the distance method. This method is usually used for diagnostics where a certain overview of the zone of interest and its boundary area is required, e.g. for the optical detection of cancer.

2.3.1 Surgical handpieces and contact tips

In the case of contact methods, the end face of an optical fibre is usually equipped with metal end caps or contact tips. Metal end caps are also known as ferrules and sometimes also referred to as heater probes or hot tips. The latter terms describe the functional principle of this type of terminal unit: the laser power transmitted by the fibre is absorbed within the metallic cap which is consequently heated. This device is applied to stop massive gastrointestinal bleeding by coagulation[22]. As shown in figure 2.11, such end caps are available with or without a laser beam outlet port. In the first case, a fraction of the laser irradiation can be used for additional tasks, whereas in the second case the complete laser power is converted into heat.

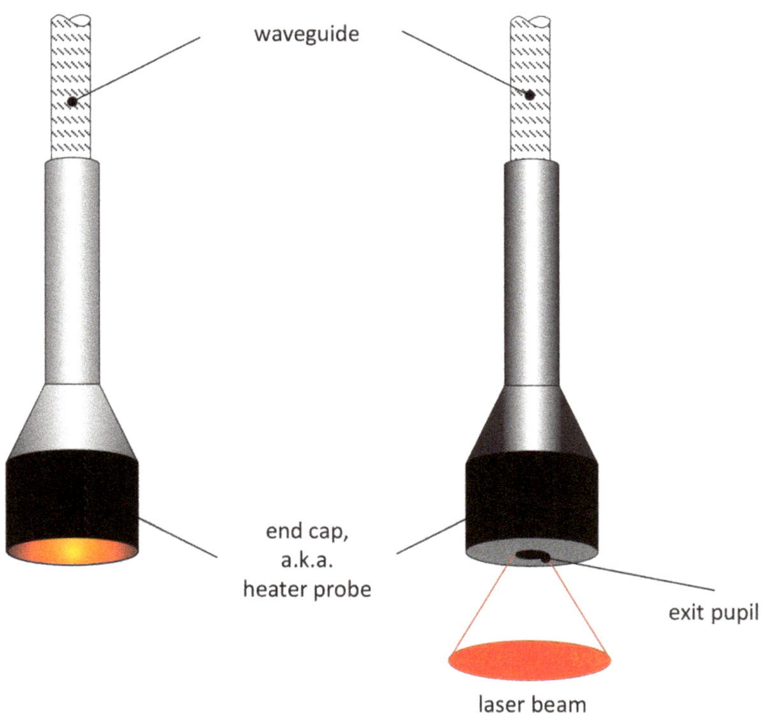

Figure 2.11. Fibre tip with metal end cap without (left) and with laser beam outlet port (right).

[22] This method is also known as heater probe coagulation (HPC). Alternatively, argon plasma coagulation (APC) is sometimes applied to stop gastrointestinal bleeding.

In contrast to metal end caps, the function of contact tips is to shape the laser beam which exits the fibre end face. The laser beam shape then mainly depends on the geometry of the transparent contact tip which is usually made of sapphire due to the advantageous properties of this optical medium[23]. Such tips are fixed on the fibre end face by a metallic connector. As shown in figure 2.12, there are three main types of contact tips, angled, plane, and spherically-shaped ones, which feature different directional characteristics.

Angled tips deliver a compressed point light source, e.g. for cutting tissue via direct contact, whereas spherically-shaped tips allow the generation of an extended point light source for large-scale and homogeneous illumination or treatment, respectively. A plane tip realises an almost collimated laser beam which is suitable for coagulation processes. The diameter of contact tips is marginally larger than the outer diameter of the fibre, i.e. hundreds of microns to a number of millimetres. Such contact tips can thus be used for both, intravascular minimal-invasive microsurgery and invasive freehand surgery. Moreover, angled fibre end faces allow extra- and intravascular treatment of tissue at defined angles of radiation. Some examples of possible applications of fibre contact tips are shown in figure 2.13.

For special applications optical fibres are used without any end cap or contact tip and even the removal of the cladding at the fibre end is applied for realising medical-optical terminal units. This approach is referred to as bare fibre technology.

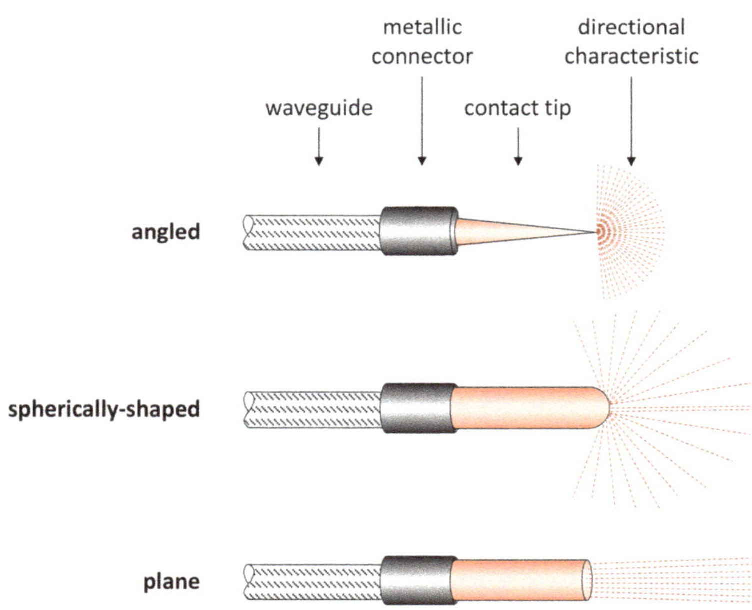

Figure 2.12. Different types of fibre contact tips including the particular directional characteristic.

[23] Sapphire stands out due to its large range of transparency from approximately 170 nm to 5.5 μm, its high index of refraction as well as chemical and mechanical resistance, and its low coefficient of thermal expansion and high thermal conductivity.

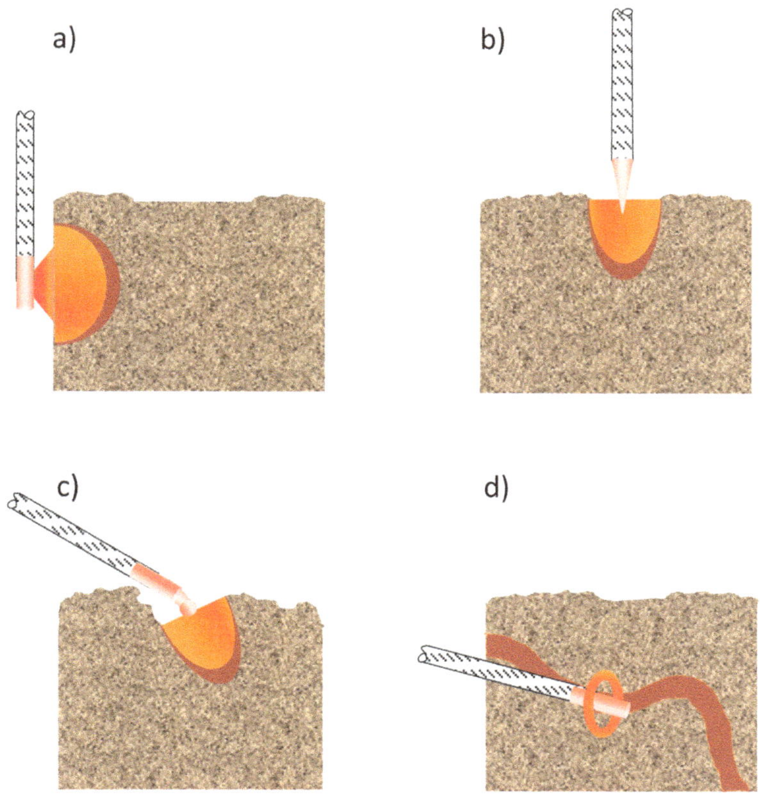

Figure 2.13. Examples for the application of fibres with contact tips; large-scale vaporisation and coagulation by the so-called side fire fibre (a), precise cutting by an angled fibre tip (b) or an angled fibre end face without any tip (c) and intravascular coagulation of inner vessel walls (d).

Applying such a bare fibre to tissue initially results in the formation of a confined and homogeneous carbonisation zone. Subsequently, the incident laser irradiation is efficiently absorbed within the carbonised zone, leading to local vaporisation and consequent removal of the tissue. The penetration depth of the laser irradiation is thus minimised and near-surface treatment is achieved.

2.3.2 Endoscopes

In modern medical diagnostic and therapy nearly all available types of flexible and rigid endoscopes are used as the terminal unit of a medical laser system where fibres are applied for the transport of laser light in most cases. The only condition for the use of an endoscope in combination with a laser apparatus is the presence of a further and sufficiently dimensioned probe channel for the following reason: rigid endoscopes contain an imaging rod lens inversion system which features high absorption of laser light and further impacts the laser beam quality. In the case of flexible endoscopes which normally contain a fibre bundle consisting of at least two single optical fibres, as shown in figure 2.14, one fibre has the function of

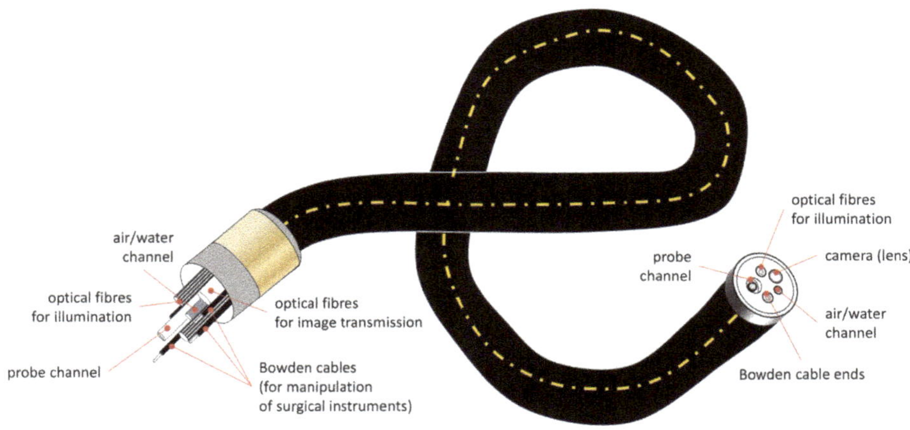

Figure 2.14. Basic setup of a flexible endoscope consisting of a bundle of different fibres with different functions.

transporting light for illumination and the other one transfers the image of the zone of interest for diagnostics or monitoring the operating field. These fibres are thus designed for such applications, but not primarily for the transportation of laser light.

In practice, illumination and monitoring are essential during the application of laser irradiation. The above-mentioned additional probe channel and the separation of the observation line from the laser beam guidance line are thus crucial. Such separation opens further possibilities for adjustment, for example by moving the laser beam-guiding fibre in order to adjust the radiant flux density in the operating field.

However, the applicability of flexible endoscopes is limited to selected laser sources due to the flexible waveguides used, i.e. optical fibres, which feature a certain transmission range as presented in more detail in section 2.2.2. In particular, infrared light is completely absorbed in any optical material commonly used for fibre cores. This avoids the guidance of CO_2 laser irradiation at a wavelength of 10.6 μm which represents an important laser source in surgery due to the fact that tissue and bones exhibit high near-surface absorption at this wavelength. Flexible fibres for this wavelength are currently developed, but not yet commercially available. Therefore, rigid endoscopes are usually used where beam guidance is obtained by reflection at the inner surface of mirror-coated tubes or channels with a manageable amount of refractive optical elements for beam expansion and focussing. Figure 2.15 shows an example of such a rigid CO_2 laser endoscope, a bronchoscope used for cutting pulmonary tissue.

Here, the actual cutting laser beam, i.e. the CO_2 laser beam, and the observation beam path, usually employing visible light, are combined with the aid of a so-called dichroic mirror. This optical element can basically be described as a low pass or high pass filter which features high transparency for one of the involved wavelengths, but high reflectivity for the other one. This allows two light beams of different wavelengths which subsequently propagate along a common path to be superimposed. Moreover, a bronchoscope exhibits several mechanical or electromechanical elements for fine adjustment of the position and the focus diameter[24] of the cutting laser beam. In order to avoid damage of optical elements due to absorption of the CO_2 laser beam at condensed moisture films on the lens or mirror surfaces, a bronchoscope tube and housing is usually flushed with air or nitrogen.

2.3.3 Operating and surgical microscopes

In order to allow the visual inspection and detection of the smallest features and objects, an optical fibre or medical endoscope may be connected to an optical microscope. Such a microscope allows the therapist or surgeon to perform actions on a very small scale such as for example required for microsurgery. These microscopes are thus referred to as operating microscope or surgical microscope. The basic setup of an optical microscope including the essential light paths is shown in figure 2.16.

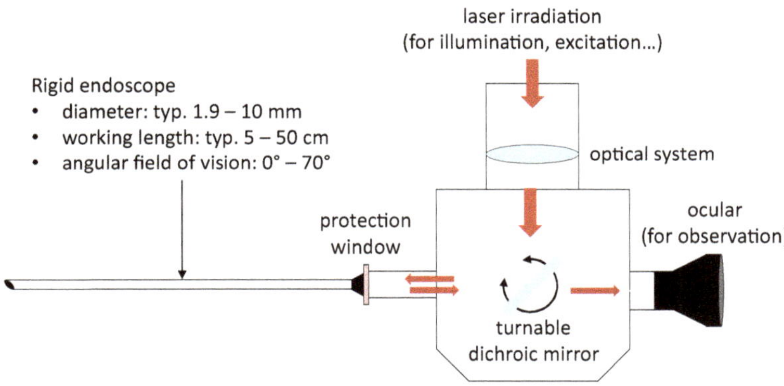

Figure 2.15. Scheme of a rigid CO_2 laser endoscope (adapted from [1]).

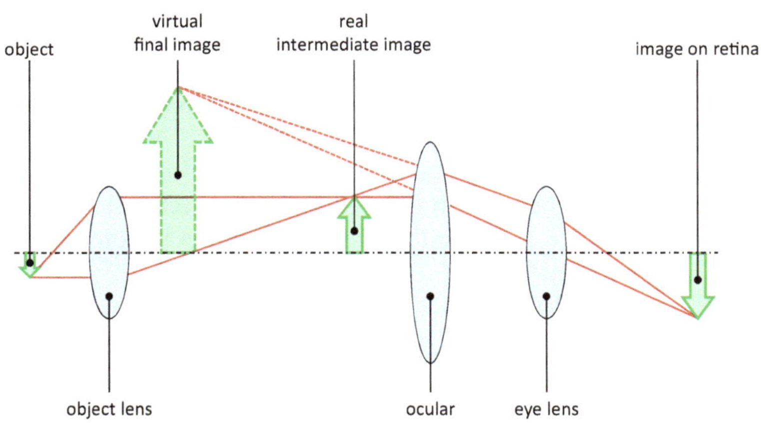

Figure 2.16. Setup of an optical microscope including the essential light paths.

[24] The focus diameter can easily be varied by increasing or decreasing the beam diameter of a collimated laser beam before focussing since the focus beam diameter is directly related to the raw beam diameter in front of the focussing optical element. In practice, this is realised by a simple adjustable telescope setup.

An object is imaged by an object lens, leading to a real intermediate image. This intermediate image is then further imaged onto the observer's retina by the optical system consisting of the microscope ocular and the observer's eye lens[25]. Consequently, a magnified virtual final image is formed where the total magnification[26] of the microscope is given by the product of the partial magnification of both the object lens and the ocular. Operating or surgical microscopes may further be equipped with special light sources for the illumination of the area of interest, for example for inducing fluorescence of labels and proteins. These systems are of outstanding importance in modern biophotonics and diagnostics such as cancer research where short-lived fluorophores are employed for the detection of cancer cells. Regarding therapeutic applications, microscopes are widely used in plastic, ophthalmic, and endodontic surgery and are essential devices in otorhinolaryngology[27] and neurosurgery.

2.4 Medical laser systems—the bottom line

- Medical laser systems normally consist of a laser source and different optical and peripheral devices as well as several control units.
- Laser light transportation from a laser system to the operating field or zone of interest for diagnosis is achieved by laser beam guidance systems or via an open beam path in a few cases.
- Mirror-based jointed arms allow the transportation of laser irradiation with wavelengths in the far ultraviolet and infrared range.
- Optical waveguides, i.e. fibres, are restricted to the visible and near infrared wavelength range due to the spectral absorption characteristics of the used optical bulk material.
- Optical fibres stand out due to extremely low diameters in the range of some hundreds of microns to a number of millimetres and the resulting high flexibility and possibility of minimally invasive intravascular application of laser light.
- Optical fibres can be classified into two main types, step index fibres and gradient index fibres, where the first type is frequently used for medical purposes.
- Step index fibres consist of a core and a cladding; both are made of transparent optical media with different indices of refraction.
- The transport of light in step index fibres is based on the physical mechanism of total internal reflection.
- The field of view of step index fibres is expressed by the fibre's numerical aperture.
- The numerical aperture of a fibre can be influenced by the index of refraction of the surrounding medium, e.g. by the use of immersion liquids as also applied in microscopy.

[25] For camera-coupled systems, the eye lens is replaced by the imaging optics of the camera used.

[26] The typical magnification of an operating or surgical microscope amounts to 4–40×.

[27] Otorhinolaryngology is the generic term for ear, nose and throat surgery, commonly abbreviated ENT surgery.

- Optical fibres are subject to different loss mechanisms such as internal damping due to absorption as well as bending losses.
- Depending on the application, a large variety of different optical terminal units and accessories is in hand.
- Heating or coagulation of tissue can be achieved by different surgical handpieces and contact tips.
- Specially-shaped end tips allow the realisation of different directional characteristics of laser light and the irradiated zone, respectively.
- Carbonisation of tissue is mainly realised with the use of bare fibres.
- Endoscopes can be classified into two main categories, rigid and flexible endoscopes.
- The applicability of flexible endoscopes in terms of the usable laser wavelengths is restricted by the transmission range of available optical fibres.
- Endoscopes contain a number of different fibres for laser beam guidance as well as simultaneous illumination and monitoring or observation.
- Operation microscopes allow monitoring microsurgical intravascular interventions or detecting smallest modifications of tissue such as cancer at its very early stage.

References

[1] Berlien H P and Müller G 2000 *Angewandte Lasermedizin—Lehr und Handbuch für Praxis und Klinik* 3rd edn (Berlin: Laser- und Medizin-Technologie) ISBN 3-609-70510-8

[2] Lutzke D 1986 *Licht Wellenleiter Technik: Bauelemente, Systeme, Messtechnik* (Dayton, USA: Pflaum)

[3] Gloge D 1972 *Appl. Opt.* **11** 2506–13

[4] Winkler C, Love J D and Ghatak A K 1979 *Opt. Quantum Electron.* **11** 173–83

[5] Kahlow H A, Kath W L and Kriegsmann G A 1991 *Bending Losses in Optical Fibers* (Boston, MA: Springer), pp 309–16 ISBN 978-1-4757-0435-8

[6] Artjushenko V G, Bukreev V S, Konov V I and Prokhorov A M 1989 *Lasers Med. Sci.* **4** 143

[7] Weber H P and Hodel W 1986 High power light-transmission in optical wavequides *High Power Lasers and Their Industrial Applications, Proc. SPIE* **650** 102–9

[8] Taylor R, Leopold K E, Mihailov S and Brimacombe R 1987 *Opt. Commun.* **63** 26–31

[9] Sowada U, Kahlert H and Basting D 1988 *Laser Optoelektron.* **20** 69

IOP Publishing

Lasers in Medical Diagnosis and Therapy

Basics, applications and future prospects

Stephan Wieneke and Christoph Gerhard

Chapter 3

Tissue optics and laser–tissue interactions

In this Chapter, the basic optical properties of biological tissue, i.e., refraction, reflexion, absorption and scattering, as well as different approaches for modelling the distribution of light within tissue are introduced. Moreover, the thermal properties of tissue are discussed and mechanisms of heat storage, conduction and dissipation are explained. Further, basic interactions of laser irradiation and tissue are presented. This includes the photochemical and thermal impact of laser light on tissue as well as the principles of photo-ablation, photodisruption, and plasma-induced ablation of tissue.

3.1 Introduction to tissue optics

Generally speaking, the interaction between laser irradiation and matter is a complex process where the particular laser-induced effects depend on a large number of influencing values and parameters. On the one hand, the actual laser parameters, i.e. the laser wavelength, its power or energy and power density or energy density, respectively, as well as—in the case of pulsed laser irradiation—the pulse duration, the pulse repetition rate, and the total applied laser dose have to be chosen carefully. On the other hand, characteristic properties of the 'work piece', i.e. mainly human tissue (or bones in some cases) in laser medicine and surgery have to be considered and the above-mentioned laser parameters have to be adapted to the specific application. Since tissue is not an optically homogeneous and isotropic medium, the interactions between laser irradiation and tissue are based on both optical and thermal mechanisms. The properties of tissue can thus be classified into two main categories: optical properties and thermal properties, as introduced in the following sections.

3.1.1 Optical properties of biological tissue

The optical properties of biological tissue are of essential importance for the description of laser-induced effects. This is due to the fact that the specific

doi:10.1088/978-0-7503-1275-2ch3

distribution of laser light within the irradiated volume follows from different optical phenomena such as refraction, reflection, absorption and scattering, as shown in figure 3.1. It thus becomes crucial to get an overview of these phenomena in order to understand the impact of laser light on tissue.

The interface between the surrounding medium, e.g. air, and tissue represents an optical interface due to the difference in index of refraction of both involved media. Such a difference in index of refraction gives rise to two main effects, reflection and refraction. Once the incident light has passed the interface and entered the tissue bulk material it is subject to scattering and absorption where the first effect is of special interest. Scattering occurs at microstructures (e.g. sebaceous glands) or particles and gives rise to a change of the direction of the propagation of light. It thus strongly impacts the distribution of light within an irradiated volume. In addition to a change in direction of propagation, a certain fraction of transmitted light may also be diffusively backscattered towards the surface and leave the irradiated volume. This effect is referred to as remission[1] and has to be distinguished from pure reflection at the surface. Finally, the conversion of light (photon energy) into heat (thermal energy) results from absorption which is thus the key mechanism for therapeutic or

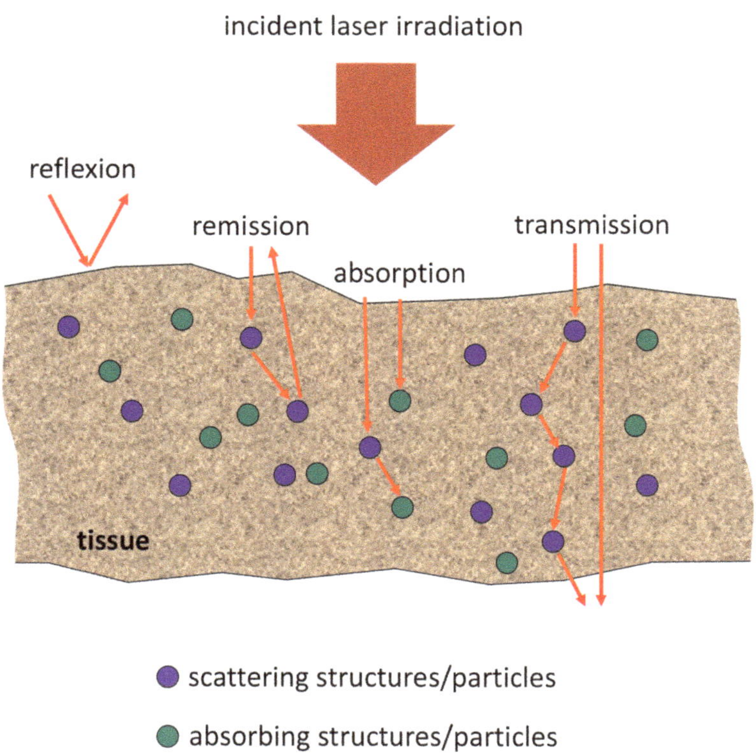

Figure 3.1. Overview of optical effects in tissue subject to laser irradiation (adapted from [1]).

[1] The fraction of light lost by remission processes within tissue can reach up to 60% in the case of near infrared laser irradiation.

surgical applications. Directly measurable (so-called macroscopic) optical properties are reflection and transmission[2] where the reflected signal consists of a fraction which results from pure surface reflection and another one which follows from remission. As shown in figure 3.2, scattering further contributes to the intensity of the transmitted signal which is further strongly dependent on the thickness of the measured sample. Scattering thus gives rise to both diffuse reflection and transmission.

When considering the initial intensity of the incident light I_0 as well as both the specular and diffuse fractions of reflected light, I_R and I_{RS}, where the index 'S' denotes scattered light, the total reflectance R can be defined according to

$$R = \frac{I_R + I_{RS}}{I_0}. \tag{3.1}$$

This relationship also applies for the total transmittance T, given by

$$T = \frac{I_T + I_{TS}}{I_0}. \tag{3.2}$$

The total absorbance A of an inhomogeneous optical medium such as tissue is finally given by

$$A = \frac{I_0 - I_R - I_{RS} - I_T - I_{TS}}{I_0}. \tag{3.3}$$

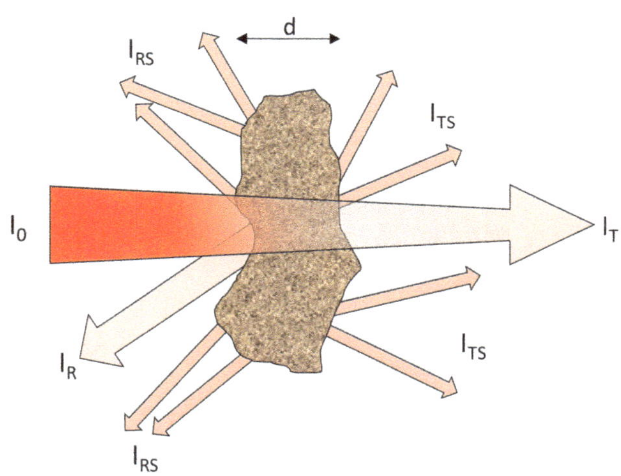

Figure 3.2. Visualisation of directly measurable optical properties of a transparent medium; incident light with the intensity I_0 is partially reflected and partially transmitted where both fractions of light are subject to specular (I_R and I_T) and diffuse (I_{RS} and I_{TS}) reflection and transmission. Note that transmission depends on the thickness d of the irradiated medium.

[2] The measurement of reflection and transmission is usually performed with the aid of UV–VIS–NIR spectrometers which allow a fast overview of the reflection and transmission characteristics of any sample within this wavelength range (approximately 190 nm to 3.5 μm, depending on the spectrometer setup and the light sources involved).

These characteristic optical properties are presented in more detail in the following sections.

Refraction

When striking an interface between two optical media with different indices of refraction, an incoming light or laser beam is subject to refraction. Such interfaces are also referred to as optical interfaces where two cases may occur: first, the incoming beam comes from an optically thin medium with the index of refraction n_1 and enters an optically denser medium with the index of refraction n_2 and second, vice versa. The first case is the normal case since usually light propagates in air ($n_{\text{air}} \approx 1$) and then enters an optically denser medium such as water ($n_{\text{water}} \approx 1.33$), glass ($n_{\text{glass}} \approx 1.45$–$1.80$) or—with respect to medical applications—tissue ($n_{\text{tissue}} \approx 1.38$). As shown in figure 3.3, the incoming light beam then changes its direction of propagation and is refracted towards its axis of incidence. This means that for each angle of incidence α_1, a specific refraction angle α_2 results. The relationship between the indices of refraction and the angle of incidence and angle of refraction, respectively, is quantified by Snell's law according to

$$\sin\alpha_1 \cdot n_1 = \sin\alpha_2 \cdot n_2. \tag{3.4}$$

Since human tissue is an optically inhomogeneous medium, its index of refraction cannot be specified as accurately as for glasses or other homogeneous optical media. However, tissue mainly consists of water, as listed in table 3.1. Its index of refraction thus correlates quite well with the index of refraction of water which can be used as an approximation, as shown in figure 3.4

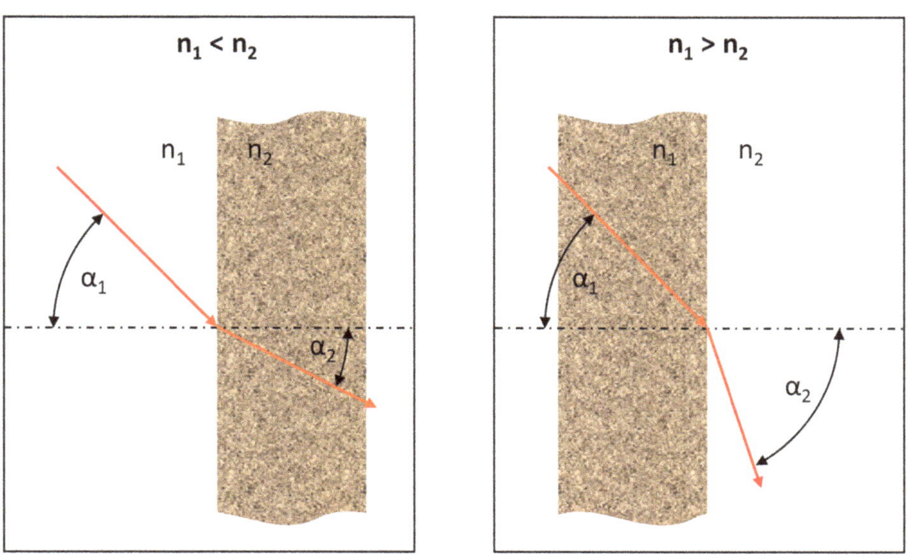

Figure 3.3. Visualisation of Snell's law, for a detailed description see the text.

Table 3.1. Overview of the water content of different organs and components of the human body.

Organ/component	Water content in %
Eye (vitreous body)	98
Blood plasma	90–95
Brain	85
Liver	77–85
Lung	84
Kidney	83–84
Blood	83
Heart	75
Muscles	75
Tissue	70
Bones	22
Hair	10

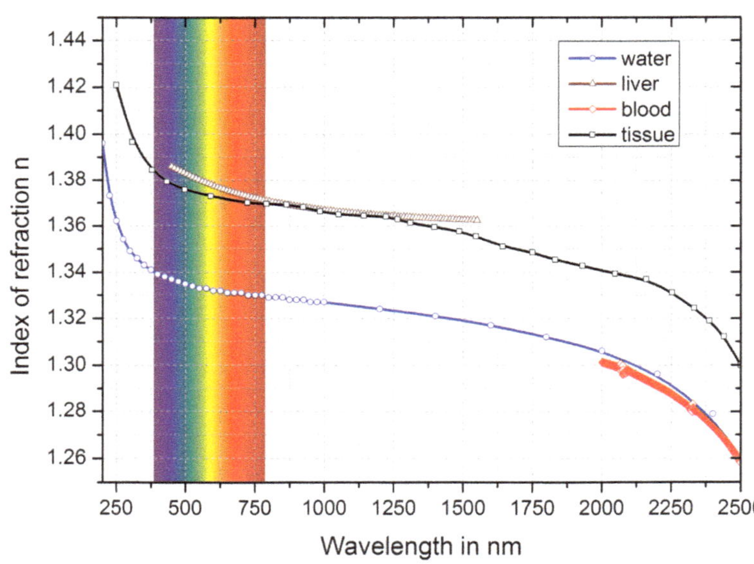

Figure 3.4. Comparison of the index of refraction of tissue, liver, blood and water versus wavelength (data taken from [2–4]).

Reflection

Another consequence of the difference in indices of refraction at optical interfaces is reflection. A high difference in the index of refraction leads to a high reflectivity of a surface[3] which is usually quantified by the reflectance R. This parameter depends on

[3] For instance, the difference in the index of refraction at an air–silver interface amounts to approximately 1.3 in the visible wavelength range. It thus features high reflectivity, whereas the surface of a window pane exhibits comparatively poor reflectivity since the difference in the index of refraction of air–glass is merely 0.2.

a number of influencing values, i.e. the wavelength[4] and polarisation of light as well as its angle of incidence on the interface. This dependence is described by the so-called Fresnel equations which allow the calculation of the particular reflectance for each polarisation state, either s-polarised or p-polarised[5], according to

$$R_{s-pol} = \left| \frac{n_1 \cdot \cos\alpha_1 - n_2 \cdot \cos\alpha_2}{n_1 \cdot \cos\alpha_1 + n_2 \cdot \cos\alpha_2} \right|^2 \tag{3.5}$$

and

$$R_{p-pol} = \left| \frac{n_2 \cdot \cos\alpha_1 - n_1 \cdot \cos\alpha_2}{n_2 \cdot \cos\alpha_1 + n_1 \cdot \cos\alpha_2} \right|^2. \tag{3.6}$$

The total reflectance R_{tot} is then given by the arithmetic mean of both fractions:

$$R_{tot} = \frac{R_{s-pol} + R_{p-pol}}{2}. \tag{3.7}$$

A special case is found for the perpendicular incidence of light where the angle of incidence amounts to 0°. Its cosine (as well as the cosine of the angle of refraction) then becomes 1, resulting in a simplified equation for the total reflectance given by

$$R_{tot} = \left(\frac{n_2 - n_1}{n_2 + n_1} \right)^2. \tag{3.8}$$

To give an approximation, the total reflectance at the interface from air to human tissue amounts to 4–60%. This wide range of possible reflectance is not only a result of different angles of incidence and the wavelength-dependence of the indices of refraction, but can also be attributed to skin type and skin pigmentation, as shown in figure 3.5.

Finally, the knowledge of the mechanisms of surface reflection and the physical characteristics involved allows the determination of the fraction of light which passes through an optical interface. The amount of transmitted light is described by the transmittance T. This parameter depends on the same influencing values as the reflectance and has thus to be calculated for each polarisation state according to

$$T_{s-pol} = \left| \frac{2 \cdot n_1 \cdot \cos\alpha_1}{n_1 \cdot \cos\alpha_1 + n_2 \cdot \cos\alpha_2} \right|^2 \tag{3.9}$$

and

---

[4] Note that the reflectance directly follows from the index of refraction which is also wavelength-dependent. This relationship is referred to as dispersion.

[5] Polarisation describes the oscillation direction of the electric field vector of an electro-magnetic wave such as laser light. Light which oscillates perpendicularly to the plane of incidence is referred to as orthogonal polarised light (abbreviated as s-polarised, from the German 'senkrecht' = 'perpendicular, orthogonal'), whereas the electric field of parallel polarised light (abbreviated as p-polarised) oscillates parallel to the plane of incidence.

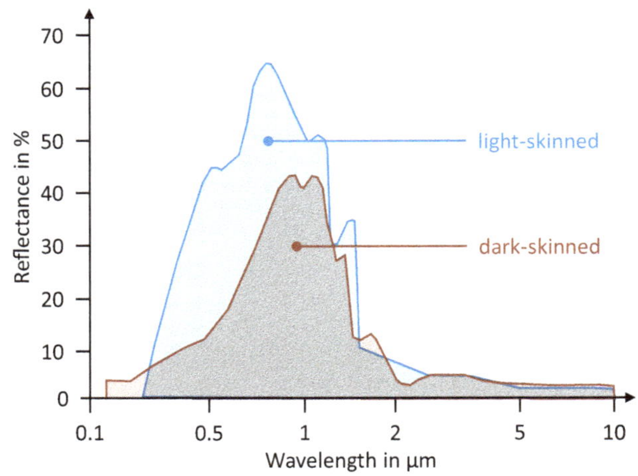

Figure 3.5. Reflectance of different skin types versus wavelength. Note that the *x*-axis is not scaled linearly (adapted from [5]).

$$T_{\text{p-pol}} = \left| \frac{2 \cdot n_1 \cdot \cos \alpha_1}{n_2 \cdot \cos \alpha_1 + n_1 \cdot \cos \alpha_2} \right|^2. \tag{3.10}$$

The total transmittance is also determined by the arithmetic mean of both fractions. Once light has passed the optical interface, it enters the bulk material and is subject to two other optical effects, absorption and scattering.

Absorption

Absorption is defined as the loss of light intensity within a medium due to the conversion of light energy into heat energy. In tissue, it can generally occur at any molecular component. Since the absorption of a medium is directly related to its index of refraction, absorption is also strongly wavelength-dependent. In the ultraviolet and visible wavelength range, different chromophores or chromophoric groups, as listed in table 3.2, act as absorbing component where the grade of absorption depends on the composition of tissue.

Within such substances, electronic transitions are excited, leading to the formation of discrete and intense absorption bands. In contrast, proteins normally feature broadened absorption bands. A quite different absorption mechanism is found in the near and mid-infrared wavelength range. Here, absorption of tissue is dominated by the absorption characteristics of water where the maximum is found at a wavelength of approximately 5 µm.

In physics, absorption is quantified by the absorption coefficient μ_a. This parameter is given by the product of the absorber concentration c_a, given in cm^{-3}, and the absorption cross section σ_a, given in cm^2, according to

$$\mu_a = \sum c_a \sigma_a. \tag{3.11}$$

Table 3.2. Selection of chromophores and chromophoric groups in tissue, acting as absorbers in the ultraviolet and visible wavelength range.

Chromophore/chromophoric group	Commentary
Porphyrin	Porphyrins are organic-chemical colourants consisting of four pyrrole rings which are interconnected via methine bridges.
Haemoglobin	Haemoglobin is a ferrous protein complex consisting of four globins. It is the reason for the red colour of blood and could be referred to as 'blood colourant'.
Melanin	Melanin is the generic term for natural pigments such as eumelanin, pheomelanin, and neuromelanin.
Flavin	Flavins are yellowish organic compounds which act as colourants. A well-known flavin is riboflavin, i.e. vitamin B_2.
Retinol	Retinol is the liposoluble vitamin A_1.
Ribonucleic acid (RNA)	RNA is a nucleic acid consisting of monomeric nucleotides. These nucleotides are composed of a pentose, a phosphate group, and a nitrogenous base.
Reduced nicotinamide adenine dinucleotide (NADH)	Nicotinamide adenine dinucleotide (NAD) is a coenzyme, its reduced form NADH features a decreased oxidation state in comparison to pure NAD.

The absorption coefficient's unit is thus cm^{-1}. Due to the large variety in possible composition, biological tissue features a wide range of absorption coefficients from $0.01\ cm^{-1}$ to $100\ cm^{-1}$.[6] The absorption and scattering mechanisms with the same target material for different wavelengths are visualised in figure 3.6. The cross section is the ability of a molecule to absorb or scatter a photon of a particular wavelength, respectively photon energy[7].

The absorption coefficient allows calculation of the transmission characteristics of any medium on the basis of the Beer–Lambert law according to

$$I_T = I_0 e^{-c_a \cdot \sigma_a \cdot d} = I_0 e^{-\mu_a \cdot d} \tag{3.12}$$

Here, I_T is the intensity of transmitted light, I_0 is the initial intensity of incident light, the product of the absorber concentration c_a and the absorption cross section σ_a is the absorption coefficient μ_a, and d is the thickness of the irradiated medium. As shown by equation (3.12) and visualised in figure 3.7, absorption within a medium is thus described by an exponential decay.

It should be noted that surface reflection is not considered by the Beer–Lambert law. It thus merely allows the calculation of the internal bulk absorption of a medium, i.e. the ratio of the transmitted intensity and the initial intensity of light,

[6] For comparison, the absorption coefficient of window glass is approximately $0.08\ cm^{-1}$.

[7] In addition to the absorption and scattering cross section, there are also other interaction cross sections such as the ionisation cross section and the cross section for inelastic impact.

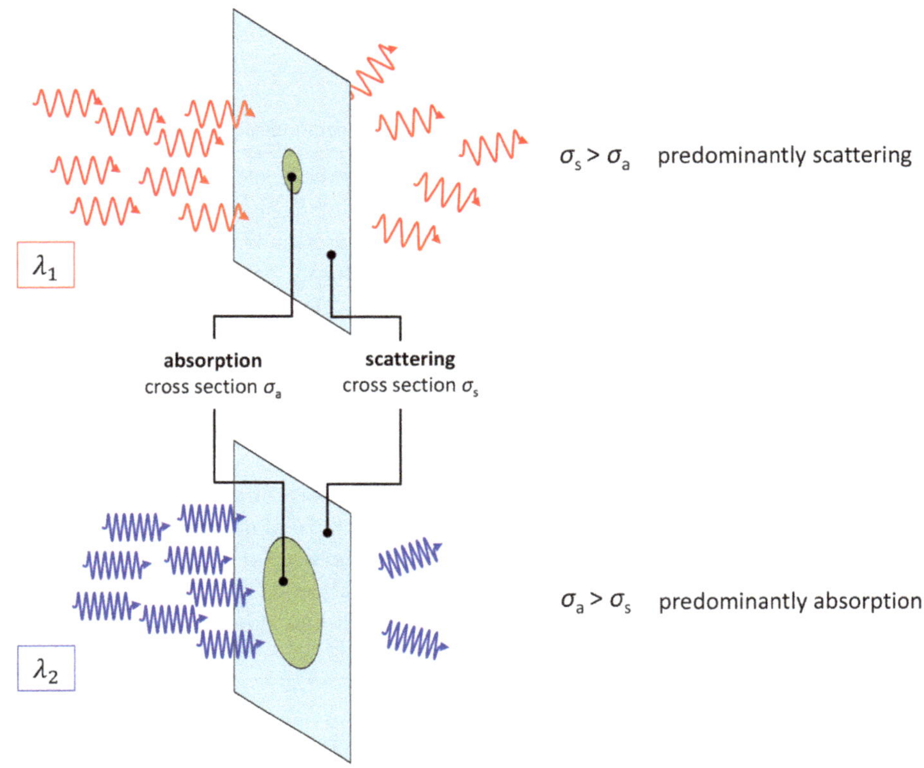

Figure 3.6. Scheme of the interaction cross sections σ_a and σ_s for scattering and absorption of incident radiation at different wavelengths.

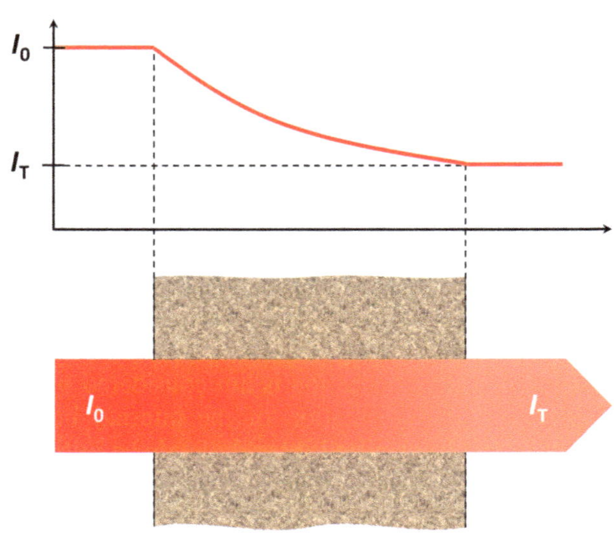

Figure 3.7. Visualisation of the decrease in light intensity I due to bulk absorption as described by the Beer–Lambert law (adapted from [6]).

I_T/I_0. In chemistry or bioanalytics, the absorption concentration c and the decade molar extinction coefficient ϵ are frequently used instead of the exponents introduced above of the Beer–Lambert law. Equation (3.12) is then rewritten as

$$I_T = I_0 \cdot 10^{-\epsilon \cdot c \cdot d} = I_0 \cdot 10^{-A} \tag{3.13}$$

The term $\epsilon \cdot c \cdot d$ is also referred to as absorbance A or optical density OD of a substance. If not otherwise specified, it refers to a sample thickness of 1 cm. Finally, it should be mentioned that the absorption coefficient μ_a and the product of the absorption concentration c and the decade molar extinction coefficient ϵ are connected by a constant according to

$$\mu_a = 2.303 \cdot c \cdot \epsilon \tag{3.14}$$

The knowledge of the absorption coefficient of any medium allows the optical depth of penetration x_{opt} of incident light to be determined easily. It is the reciprocal value of the absorption coefficient,

$$x_{opt} = \frac{1}{\mu_a} \tag{3.15}$$

and defines the mean free length of the path into the absorbing medium. The most important absorbing medium in biological tissue is water. The wavelength-dependent absorption coefficient of this medium is shown in figure 3.8. For comparison, the absorption coefficients of oxygenated human haemoglobin and further selected components of tissue are shown in figures 3.9 and 3.10, respectively.

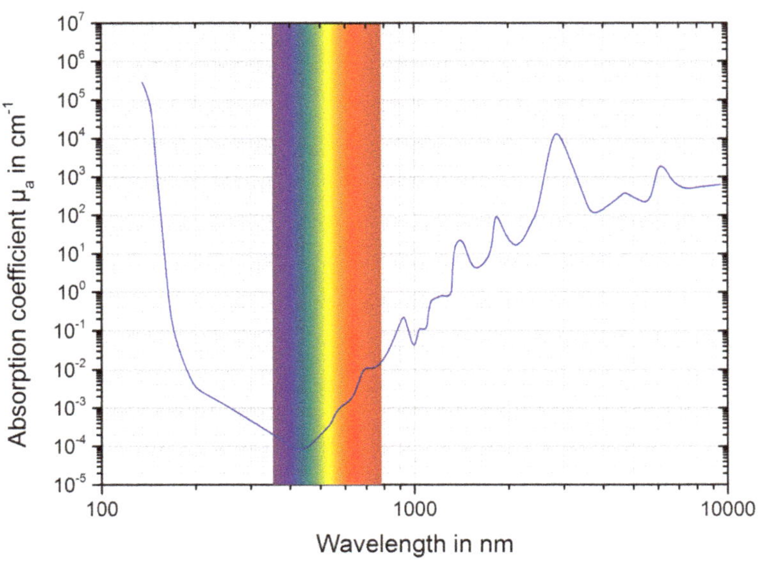

Figure 3.8. Absorption coefficient of pure water versus wavelength (adapted from [7]).

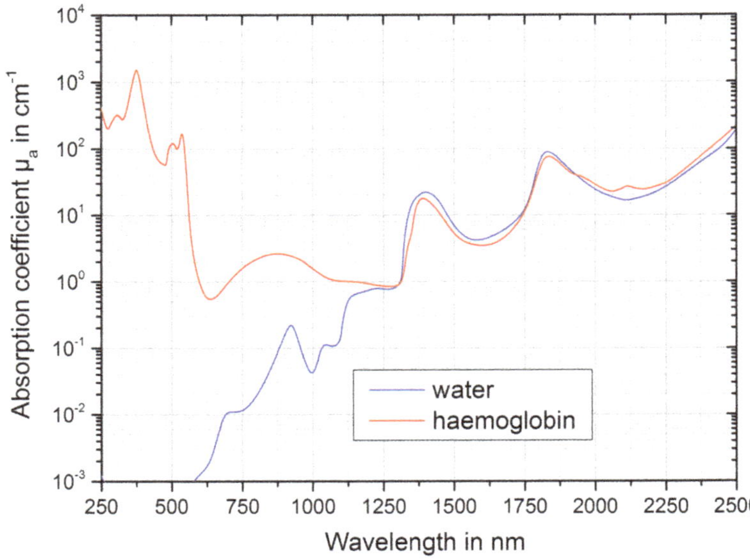

Figure 3.9. Absorption coefficient of human haemoglobin in the wavelength range 250–2500 nm.

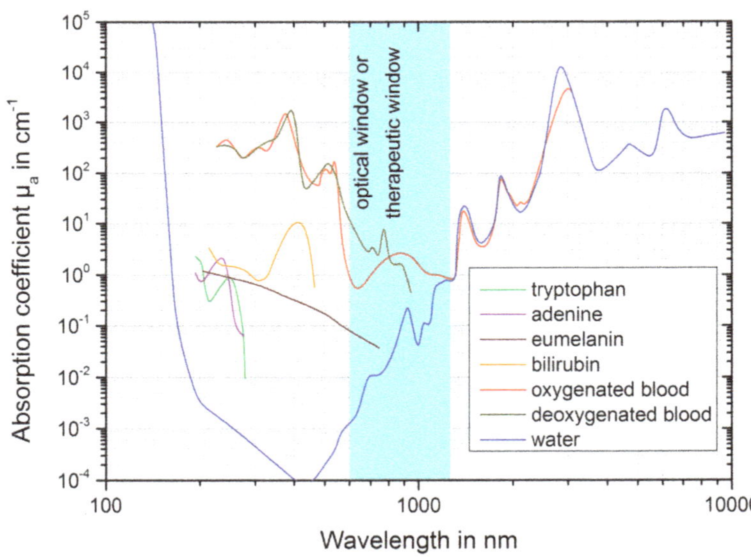

Figure 3.10. Absorption characteristics of different components of tissue versus wavelength including the so-called optical or therapeutic window in the wavelength range from approximately 600 nm to 1.2 μm.

Scattering

The distribution of light and its intensity within a certain volume of tissue is mainly determined by the tissue's scattering characteristics which results from the structure of the tissue. Scattering is defined as the change in the propagation direction of light without any loss in energy. It is thus a mechanism which occurs prior to absorption and heat generation. The phenomenon of light scattering can be classified into two main categories, Rayleigh scattering and Mie scattering. In the first case, scattering occurs at so-called microscopic structures with a lateral size d which is much smaller than the wavelength of light, $d \ll \lambda$. In contrast, scattering at macroscopic structures with a lateral size bigger than the wavelength, $d > \lambda$ is referred to as Mie scattering. For instance, muscle fibres, dermal layers or dentinal tubules are macroscopic structures, whereas cells or intracellular structures represent microscopic or even sub-microscopic[8] structures. In reality, scattering within tissue is a mixture of both types of scattering, as shown in figure 3.11, where the dominating mechanism depends on the composition of the tissue and the predominant structures and structure sizes. Scattering structures are usually referred to as scatter centres.

Rayleigh scattering is an isotropic mechanism which merely depends on the polarisation and the wavelength of light. The scattering cross section σ_s is inversely proportional to the fourth power of wavelength, λ^4. It is given by

$$\sigma_s = A \cdot Q_s \tag{3.16}$$

where A is the area of a scattering structure and Q_s is the scattering efficiency which can be determined according to

$$Q_s = \frac{128\pi^4 d^4}{3\lambda^4} \left| \frac{n_s^2 - n^2}{n_s^2 + 2n^2} \right|. \tag{3.17}$$

Here, d is the diameter of the scattering structure or particle and n_s its index of refraction, λ is the wavelength of incident light, and n is the index of refraction of the surrounding medium. In comparison to Rayleigh scattering, the calculation of Mie scattering is much more complex and is thus usually performed by so-called Monte

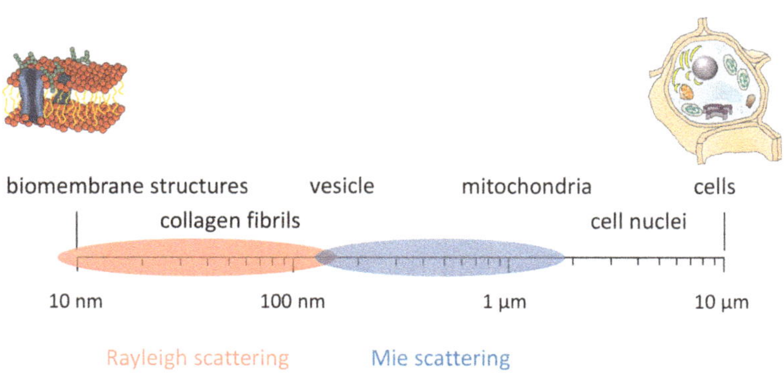

Figure 3.11. Classification of Rayleigh and Mie scattering at different tissue structures (adapted from [8]).

[8] As an example, macromolecules or nanoparticles are sub-microscopic structures with lateral sizes in the range of some tens to some hundreds of nanometres which can be found in tissue.

Carlo simulation (MCS)[9]. As shown in figure 3.12, light is predominantly forward-scattered in the case of Mie scattering.

As a result, the light which is scattered by different scatter centres is subject to constructive and destructive interference. Such interference gives rise to the formation of intensity maxima and minima when taking a closer look at the angle-dependence of scattered light, as shown in figure 3.12. This example shows the complexity of this scattering mechanism which does not exclusively include pure scattering, but also secondary effects which may arise from diffraction and interference. Scattering can generally be described by the scattering coefficient μ_s. Similar to the absorption coefficient (see equation (3.11)), this parameter is given by the product of the concentration of scatter centres c_s, given in cm^{-3}, and the scattering cross section σ_s, given in cm^2. The scattering coefficient is determined by summing scattering which occurs for different types of scatter centres according to

$$\mu_s = \sum c_s \sigma_s. \tag{3.18}$$

The reciprocal value of the scattering coefficient, $1/\mu_s$, is the mean free length of path between two scattering occurrences. The scattering coefficient thus quantifies the number of scattering occurrences per distance. For biological tissue, it is typically

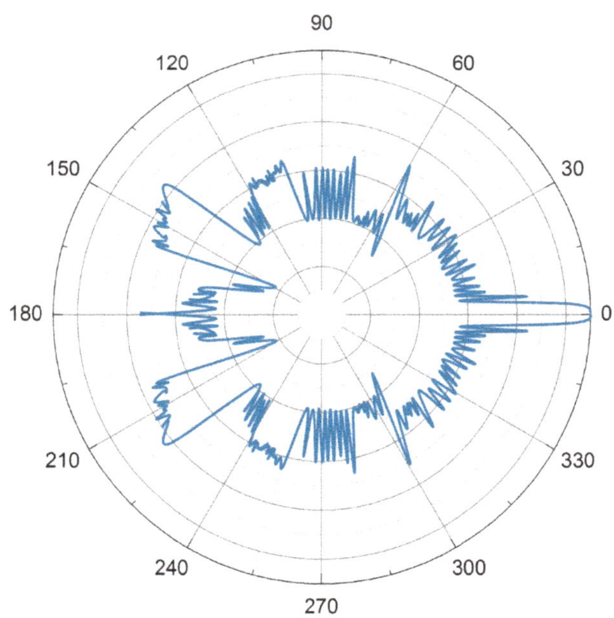

Figure 3.12. Mie scattering diagram of a water drop. This representation is given in polar coordinates where the values shown are in degrees.

[9] Computer-assisted MCS are employed for mathematical tasks, where the results depend on an extensive number of input variables, resulting in a long time required for computing. It is realised by repeating random sampling via appropriate computational algorithms.

found in the range 10–1000 cm^{-1} [9]. For a broad wavelength range, the scattering coefficient is notably higher than the absorption coefficient[10]. Its wavelength-dependence is quite moderate and can be approximated by a $1/\lambda$ function for most tissues. This means that scattering decreases with increasing wavelength, as shown in figure 3.13.

As already mentioned above, an all-encompassing mathematical description of real scattering processes is nearly impossible due to the large number and variety of scatter centres. As a consequence, scattering within biological tissue cannot be entirely characterised via the scattering coefficient, but an additional parameter which describes the angular distribution, as shown in figure 3.12, is required. The angular distribution indicates the change in propagation direction of all involved photons and is thus of great interest. It is usually specified by the so-called anisotropy factor g which is given by the mean cosine of the scattering angle θ according to

$$g = \langle \cos \theta \rangle. \tag{3.19}$$

This anisotropy factor allows the determination of the preferred direction of scattering: for $-1 < g < 0$, backscattering[11] is found, whereas forward-scattering[12]

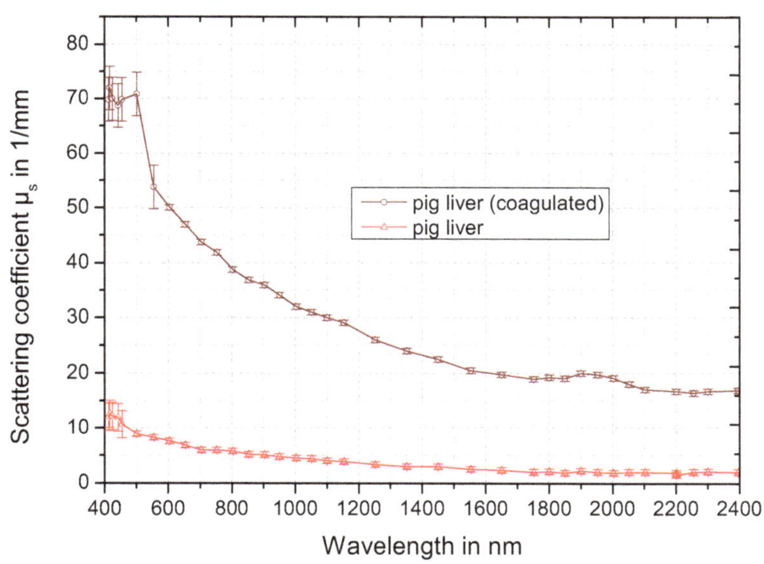

Figure 3.13. Scattering coefficient of pig liver versus wavelength (adapted from [10]).

---

[10] Within human tissue, the mean free length of path of red light is approximately 50 μm for absorption and about 5 mm for scattering. From a statistical point of view, a photon is thus scattered 100 times before it is absorbed.

[11] Backscattering is the preferred scattering of light towards its source.

[12] If light propagates preferentially along its initial direction of propagation after scattering, the effect of forward-scattering is predominant. This especially applies for Mie scattering, see figure 3.12.

occurs if $0 < g < 1$, as shown in figure 3.14. Isotropic scattering[13] is indicated by an anisotropy factor of $g = 0$.

Biological tissue normally exhibits strong forward-scattering where the anisotropy factor is found in the range from $0.8 < g < 0.99$ [9, 11] for visible and near infrared light. In tissue optics and especially for MCS, a certain probability function or dispersion phase function for g has to be taken into account. Here, different mathematical approaches are in hand where a commonly-used dispersion phase function is the so-called Henyey–Greenstein phase function[14].

This function describes the angular distribution of scattered light by the scattering probability $p(\theta)$ and is given by

$$p(\theta) = \frac{1}{4\pi}\frac{1 - g^2}{[1 + g^2 - 2g\cos(\theta)]^{3/2}}. \tag{3.20}$$

This model has turned out to be a suitable and powerful tool for the description of scattering in complex systems such as biological tissue or interstellar clouds of dust where the parameter g characterises the normalised distribution. The scattering probability for selected values of g and the angular range from $-180°$ to $+180°$ is shown in figure 3.15.

For anisotropy factors close to 1, this function exhibits a steep maximum around a scattering angle of $\theta = 0$, indicating predominant forward-scattering. For isotropic scattering, where $g = 0$, a constant value of $1/4\pi$ occurs for each scattering angle according to equation (3.20). In the case of multiple scattering, the information on the direction of arrival of light may get lost after a few scattering events. The effective phase function then becomes isotropic. It is thus helpful to average the involved scattering events and to introduce an effective scattering coefficient $\acute{\mu}_s$, given by

$$\acute{\mu}_s = \left(-\int_{4\pi} p(\theta)\cos(\theta)d\Omega\right)\mu_s = (1 - g)\mu_s. \tag{3.21}$$

This also applies for the absorption coefficient. The sum of the scattering and absorption coefficient finally gives the total attenuation factor μ_{tot}. Another

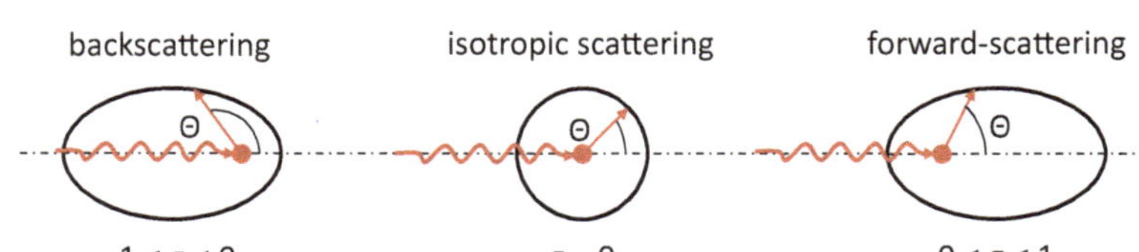

Figure 3.14. Preferred direction of scattering including the particular co-domain of the anisotropy factor g (adapted from [1]).

---

13 In the case of isotropic scattering, the distribution of scattered light is given by a concentric circle around the scatter centre.

14 The Henyey–Greenstein phase function is a probability density function (PDF), it is thus normalised to 1.

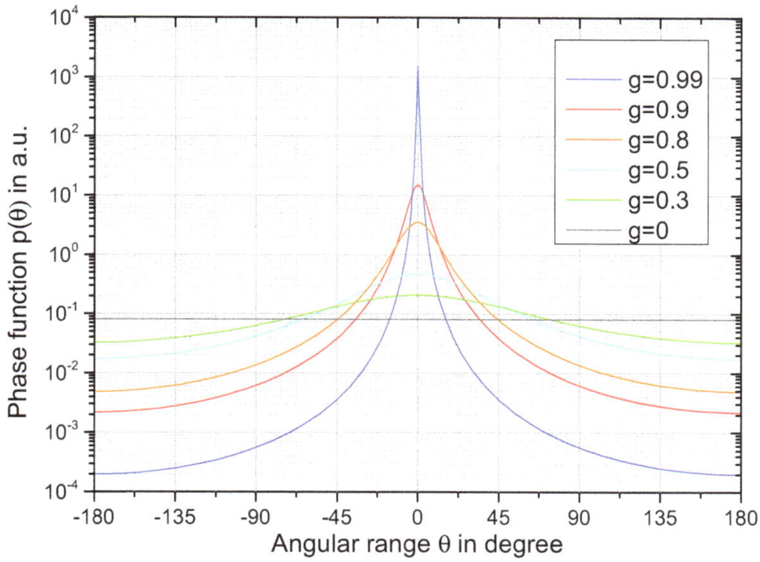

Figure 3.15. Henyey–Greenstein phase function for selected anisotropy factors g and the angular range from −180° to +180°.

parameter for the description of the optical properties of tissue is the so-called albedo a, given by

$$a = \frac{\mu_s}{(\mu_s + \mu_a)}. \tag{3.22}$$

This parameter is found in the range from 0 to 1. For $a = 0$, i.e. $\mu_s = 0$, no scattering occurs, whereas no absorption takes place for $a = 1$, which is equivalent to $\mu_a = 0$. A further helpful parameter, the effective attenuation coefficient μ_{eff} is given by

$$\mu_{eff} = \sqrt{3\mu_a(\mu_a + \acute{\mu}_s)}. \tag{3.23}$$

The reciprocal value of this attenuation coefficient is referred to as the effective optical depth of penetration $x*_{opt}$ of light,

$$x_*^{opt} = \frac{1}{\mu_{eff}}. \tag{3.24}$$

where scattering is considered additionally in contrast to the optical depth of penetration, as introduced in section 3.1.1. The effective free length of path l_{eff} then accounts for

$$l_{eff} = \frac{1}{\mu_a + \acute{\mu}_s}. \tag{3.25}$$

Tissue is a strongly scattering optical medium where the distribution of light intensity is not only determined by pure absorption according to the Beer–

Table 3.3. Overview on the nominal absorption coefficient μ_a and the related effective attenuation coefficient μ_{eff} of soft tissue as well as the corresponding nominal optical depth of penetration x_{opt} and the effective optical depth of penetration x^*_{opt}, respectively, for selected laser wavelengths in the ultraviolet, visible, and infrared wavelength range [12, 13].

λ [nm]	μ_a [cm $^{-1}$]	μ_{eff} [cm^{-1}]	x_{opt} [λm]	x^*_{opt} [λm]
193	400	5000	25	2
248	600	5000	17	2
308	200	1670	50	6
351	40	170	250	60
532	12	42	830	240
1064	4	5	2500	1900
2060	35	40	286	250
2940	3000	3000	3	3
10 600	600	$\approx$ 600	17	17

Lambert law (see equation (3.12)), but also results from scattering. This fact is taken into account and pointed out by the comparison of the nominal absorption coefficient and the related effective attenuation coefficient on the one hand and the nominal optical depth of penetration and the related effective optical depth of penetration on the other hand, as listed in table 3.3.

3.1.2 Modelling the distribution of light in biological tissue

As has already been discussed, the distribution of light in biological tissue depends on the prevailing optical effect, scattering or absorption. A strongly absorbing tissue is schematically shown in figure 3.16(a). In this example, scattering is negligible with respect to absorption and incoming light is consequently completely absorbed within a thin near-surface layer[15]. In this example, the initial laser beam intensity of $I_0 = 1$ W cm^{-2} is reduced by three orders of magnitude (to 0.001 W cm^{-2}) after passing such absorbing tissue with a thickness of merely 2 mm. This behaviour is crucial for precise laser cutting of tissue. In contrast, strong scattering, as shown in figure 3.16(b), is advantageous for a homogeneous heating of tissue as, for example, is needed for coagulation processes. Due to strong scattering and the accompanying spatial accumulation of laser light, even higher intensities than the intensity I_0 of the incident laser beam may arise within a near-surface layer, as shown by the values of the isothermal lines in figure 3.16(b).

Modelling the distribution of light in any optically inhomogeneous medium, and especially in biological tissue, is a challenging task. However, several approaches for calculating the distribution and diffusion of photons in tissue are in hand where the choice of a suitable model depends mainly on the particular values for the absorption coefficient μ_a and the effective scattering coefficient $\acute{\mu}_s$. As listed in

[15] This effect is called surface absorption and occurs for media with high absorbance A. In contrast, media with high transmittance T are subject to bulk absorption.

table 3.4, different cases including the particularly suitable model and valid wavelength range can be classified.

Modelling by the Beer–Lambert law

In the case of high absorption, the depth-dependent photon density, i.e. the intensity of light can be described by the Beer–Lambert law, as introduced in section 3.1.1. Taking the effective attenuation coefficient μ_{eff} into account, equation (3.12) can be rewritten as

$$I(d) = I_0 e^{-\mu_{eff} d} \tag{3.26}$$

In an actual measurement setup, photons could pass a certain sample thickness d and arrive on a detector after a number of scattering events. For dominating forward-scattering, the effective scattering coefficient $\acute{\mu}_s$ is much smaller than the regular scattering coefficient μ_s and some photons may have covered a significantly higher actual distance than the theoretical distance d, i.e. the sample thickness. This fact shows that for strongly scattering media such as tissue, the depth of penetration

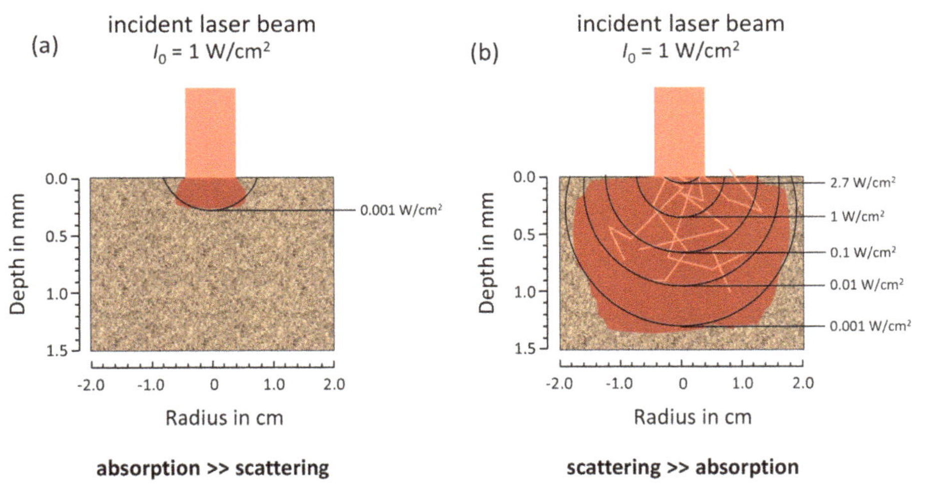

Figure 3.16. Example for the distribution of light within strongly absorbing (a) and strongly scattering (b) tissues.

Table 3.4. Different cases of relationships of the absorption coefficient μ_a and the effective scattering coefficient $\acute{\mu}_s$ including the particularly suitable model and valid wavelength range.

Case	Model	Wavelength range
$\mu_a \gg \acute{\mu}_s$	Beer–Lambert law	λ < 300 nm and λ > 2 μm
$\mu_a \ll \acute{\mu}_s$	Diffusion approximation	600 nm < λ < 1.2 μm
$\mu_a \approx \acute{\mu}_s$	Radiative transfer equation based on MCS	300 nm < λ < 650 nm and 1.15 μm < λ < 2 μm

cannot be exclusively determined on the basis of the Beer–Lambert law, as discussed above. This especially applies for the so-called optical or therapeutic window, i.e. the wavelength range from 600 nm to 1.2 μm, where cells and biological tissue feature low attenuation of light (compare figure 3.10). Here, the diffusion approximation can be used for modelling the distribution of light within tissue.

Modelling by the diffusion approximation

The diffusion approximation is an approach for describing the expansion of photons within a medium with dominating scattering characteristics. In the case of tissue, the dominance of scattering within the optical window becomes obvious when comparing the absorption coefficient ($\mu_a \approx 0.001$–$1\ \text{mm}^{-1}$) and the effective scattering coefficient ($\acute{\mu}_s \approx 1$–$10\ \text{mm}^{-1}$). Hence, photons expand in a similar way to a classical diffusion process, driven by a gradient in concentration, and according to the diffusion equation, given by

$$\left(\frac{1}{c}\frac{\partial}{\partial t} - D(r)\nabla^2 + \mu_a(r)\right)\rho(r, t) = Q_0(r, t). \tag{3.27}$$

Here, c is the speed of light within the tissue which follows from the ratio of the speed of light in vacuum c_0 and the index of refraction of the tissue n,

$$c = \frac{c_0}{n}. \tag{3.28}$$

$D(r)$ is the diffusion constant, given by

$$D(r) = \frac{1}{3}\cdot\frac{1}{\left[\mu_a(r) + [1 - g(r)]\mu_s(r)\right]}, \tag{3.29}$$

$\rho(r, t)$ is the photon density and $Q_0(r, t)$ is the source term for photons. However, this diffusion equation merely allows an approximation of the distribution of photons. An exact description is made possible by the radiative transfer equation according to

$$\begin{aligned}\frac{\partial f(r, \Omega, t)}{\partial t} = {} & Q_0(r, \Omega, t) + \mu_s(r)\int_{4\pi} p(\acute{\Omega} \to \Omega) f(r, \Omega, t)\, d\acute{\Omega} \\ & - \Omega\nabla f(r, \Omega, t) - [\mu_s(r) + \mu_a(r)] f(r, \Omega, t).\end{aligned} \tag{3.30}$$

This complex equation implies that the change in the number of photons per time interval with the direction of motion Ω which are located within a volume dV at a point of time $t + dt$ must correspond to an effective number of photons. This effective number of photons is given by the sum of the number of photons provided by the light source and the gain in photons due to scattering from the directions $\acute{\Omega}$ minus the loss in photons. This loss includes reflection at the optical interface, scattering in different directions as well as remission, and absorption within the volume dV. It turns out that solving the radiative transfer equation represents a challenging task due to the high number of variables. Here, MCS are suitable and powerful tools with high computational accuracy.

Monte Carlo simulations

In the course of an MCS, the ray paths, also known as trajectories, of a pre-defined number of photons are calculated statistically. Finally, the remission and transmission properties of an optical medium with given characteristic parameters are determined, as shown in figure 3.17.

A reversal of an MCS allows the determination of unknown optical parameters and characteristics on the basis of measured values such as for example the reflectance R and the transmittance T. In this case, simulation of the optical parameters of an optical medium with arbitrary start values for the absorption coefficient μ_a, the scattering coefficient μ_s and the anisotropy factor g are calculated and compared to the actually measured values. Moreover, an acceptable error limit for the deviation between the simulated and the measured values is defined. In the case of high deviation, a gradient matrix is determined. Then, the above-mentioned start parameters are adjusted on the basis of the gradient matrix and the simulation is rerun with these new and adapted start values. This step is repeated iteratively until the error limit for the deviation is reached or even undercut. Figure 3.18 shows the flow diagram of such a process.

Even though the determination of the reflectance R and the transmittance T of any sample is quite simple, the direct measurement of scattering and absorption is notably complex[16] and requires sophisticated approaches and equipment. As an example,

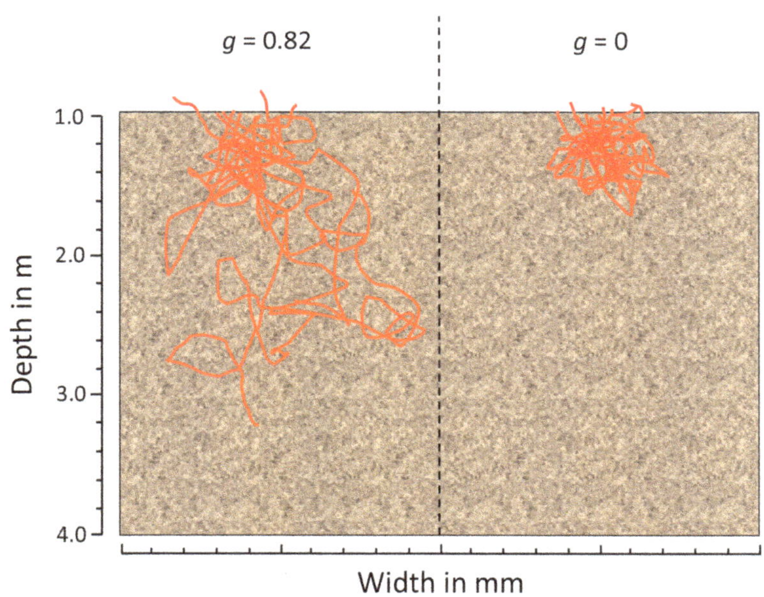

Figure 3.17. MCS of the ray paths of a number of photons (here: 10^5–10^8) within tissue (dermis, $\mu_a = 2.7$ cm^{-1}, $\mu_s = 187$ cm^{-1}) with an anisotropy factor of $g = 0.82$ (left) and $g = 0$ (right). The wavelength of light is $\lambda = 633$ nm.

[16] The detected reflected signal which gives the reflectance R may include a certain portion of remission. The separation of pure surface reflection and remission is a challenging task due to the fact that diffuse reflection at rough optical interfaces may be interpreted as a remission effect.

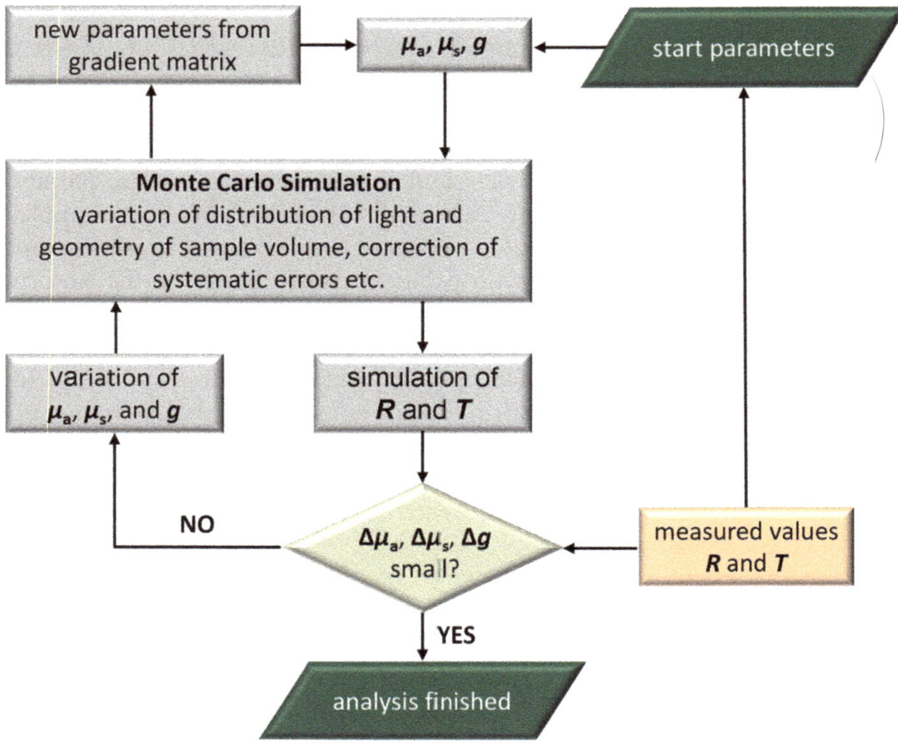

Figure 3.18. Flow diagram of an MCS process for the determination of the absorption coefficient μ_a, the scattering coefficient μ_s, and the anisotropy factor g on the basis of measured values for the reflectance R and the transmittance T (adapted from [11, 14]).

diffuse backscattering R_d and total transmission T_t of tissue samples are measured *in vitro* with the aid of integrating spheres, also known as Ulbricht spheres. In addition, the non-scattered, collimated transmission T_c is determined, as shown in figure 3.19.

The integrating spheres used feature a highly reflecting inner surface which allows the detection of the entire reflected or transmitted light at the front side and the back side of a sample. The use of broadband light sources such as mercury (Hg) or xenon (Xe) lamps and the additional use of monochromators allows the spectral analysis of the sample in a wavelength range of approximately 300 nmn to 2.5 μm. The wanted parameters μ_a, μ_s, g can finally be derived from the measured parameters R_d, T_t, and T_c. The setup shown in figure 3.19 becomes much simpler when merely a single or two parameters are to be determined, as shown in figures 3.20, 3.21, and 3.22.

Moreover, the determination of optical characteristics of tissue can be carried out by successive replacing of the sample within a single integrated sphere, as shown in figure 3.23, or with the aid of rotatable segmented integrating spheres, as shown in figure 3.24.

3.1.3 Thermal properties of biological tissue

The knowledge of the thermal properties of biological tissue becomes crucial for a description of the conversion of light energy into heat and the subsequent heat

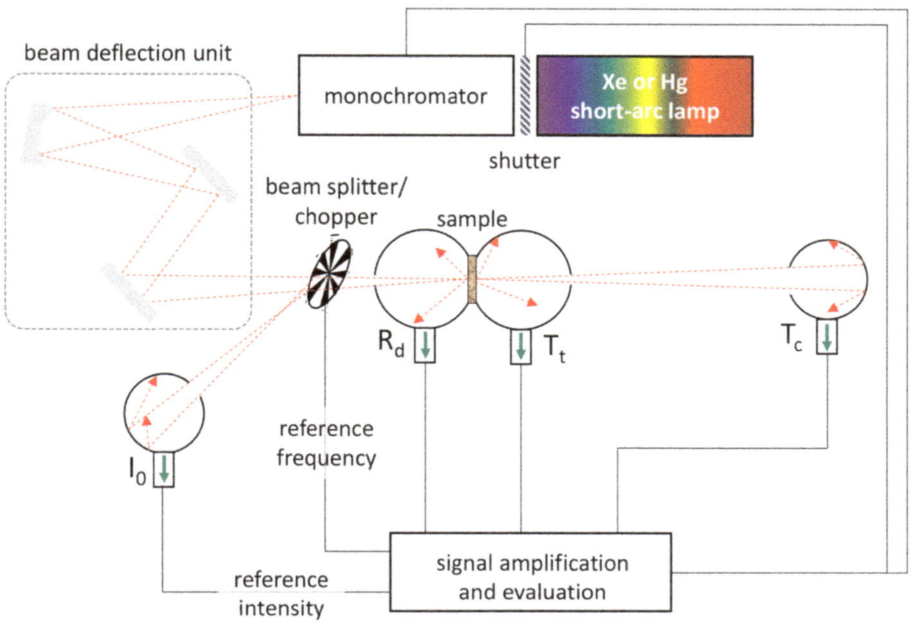

Figure 3.19. Example of a double integrating sphere measurement setup for the determination of diffuse backscattering R_{d}, total transmission T_{t}, and non-scattered, collimated transmission T_{c} (adapted from [11, 14]).

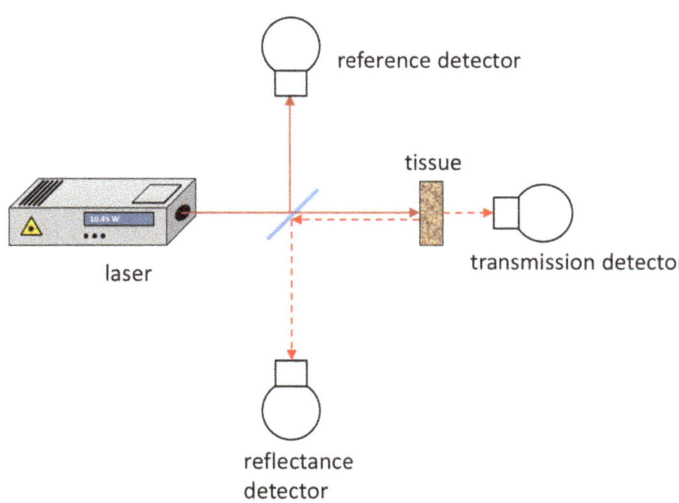

Figure 3.20. Setup for the direct measurement of transmittance and absorption (adapted from [15]).

transfer within tissue. As discussed above, the expansion of light or laser irradiation underlies different mechanisms where different optical characteristics such as reflection, transmission, scattering and absorption are involved. In contrast, the direct interaction of light and tissue is exclusively due to absorption at

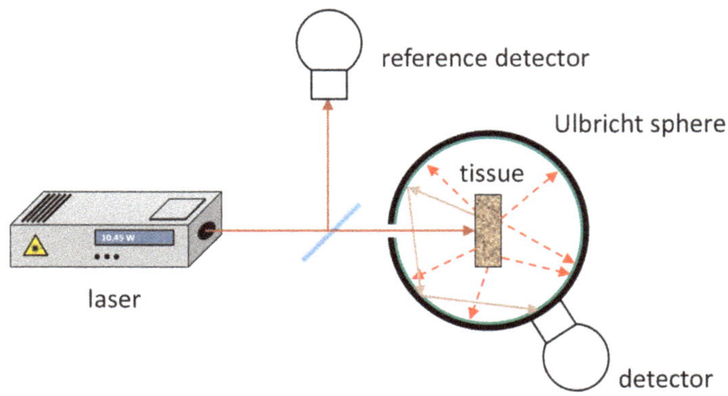

Figure 3.21. Setup for the measurement of absolute absorption (adapted from [15]).

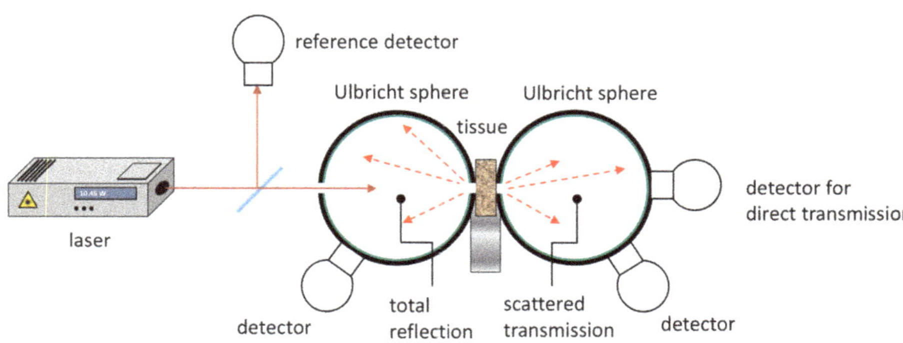

Figure 3.22. Setup for the measurement of absolute reflectance and transmittance as well as direct transmission using double integrating spheres, also known as Ulbricht spheres, for the determination of absolute absorption (adapted from [15]).

chromophores[17], as listed in table 3.2. The heat source density Q (given in W m^{-3}) within irradiated tissue is thus a function of the absorption coefficient μ_a and the total irradiance L (given in W m^{-2}). As expressed by equation (3.31), the latter parameter consists of two fraction values, the direct and collimated irradiance L_c and the scattered irradiance L_s, i.e. light deflected towards the heat source by scattering within the surrounding tissue:

$$Q(\vec{r}, t) = \mu_a \underbrace{[L_c(\vec{r}, t) + L_s(\vec{r}, t)]}_{\text{total irradiance } L}. \tag{3.31}$$

[17] Absorption and chromophoric behaviour are strongly wavelength-dependent. A chromophore is thus not necessarily visible to the naked eye. For instance, water is transparent in the visible wavelength range, but is an excellent absorber/chromophore in the infrared wavelength range, e.g. for carbon dioxide laser irradiation at a wavelength of $\lambda = 10.6$ μm

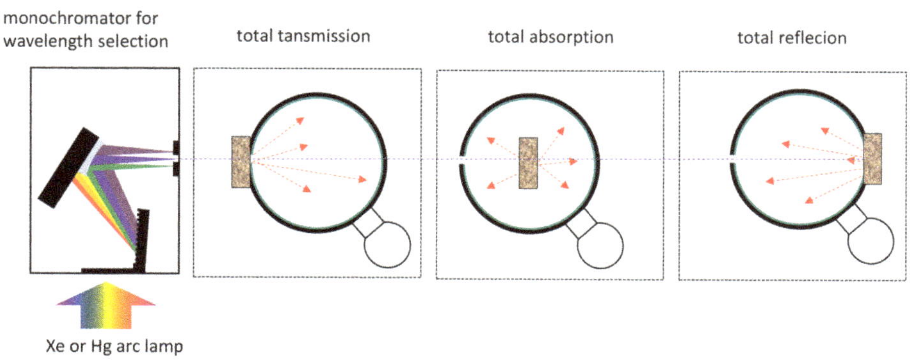

Figure 3.23. Measurement of total transmission, absorption, and reflection by successive replacing of the sample.

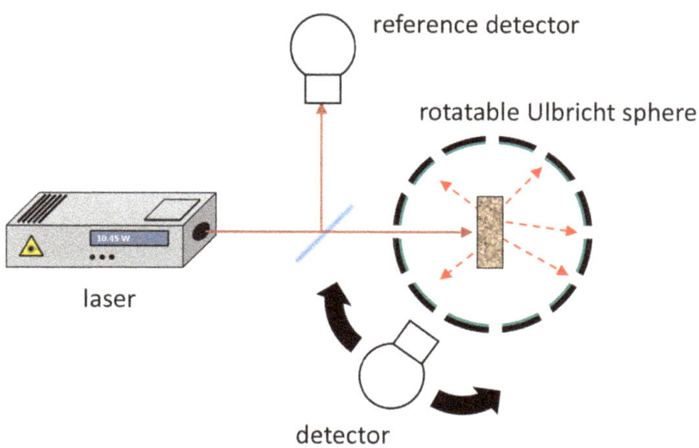

Figure 3.24. Measurement of the anisotropy factor applying a rotatable segmented integrating sphere (adapted from [15]).

The conversion of light energy into heat gives rise to a local increase in temperature within the irradiated volume. As long as no phase transition[18] takes place, the temperature T increases proportionally to the heat source density Q. As a consequence, a temperature gradient is formed and heat is transferred towards colder regions. This limits the maximum temperature of an irradiated region which is directly related to the intensity of incident light. Moreover, each type of tissue exhibits a certain intensity threshold which needs to be exceeded in order to obtain a defined local temperature. The inserted energy is partially transported to neighbouring zones of the tissue. As a consequence, not only the irradiated volume, but also its

[18] Generally, phase transition is the transition from an initial state of aggregation to another one due to either the absorption or the release of energy. In the case of phase transition on the basis of absorption of energy, this process is referred to as endothermic (in contrast to an exothermic process where energy is released, e.g. during the condensation of water vapour). Endothermic phase transitions are: solid to liquid, liquid to gaseous, gaseous to plasma state.

surroundings are heated. The thermal reactions of living tissue contributing to this effect are mainly (i) heat storage, (ii) heat conduction, and (iii) heat dissipation by blood flow, as presented in more detail in the following sections.

Heat storage

When absorbed, incoming light or irradiation causes a heating of tissue. This laser-induced heat storage and the resulting increase in temperature ΔT can be described by the inter-relationship

$$\Delta T = \frac{Q}{\rho c}. \tag{3.32}$$

Here, Q is the absorbed thermal energy per volume unit, given in J m^{-3}, ρ is the density of the tissue, given in kg m^{-3}, and c is the specific heat capacity, i.e. the heat capacity per unit mass of a material and thus given in J kg^{-1} K^{-1}. As an approximation, the specific heat capacity of tissue can be estimated according to [16, 17]

$$c = \left(1.55 + 2.8\frac{w}{\rho}\right)\left[\frac{\mathrm{kJ}}{\mathrm{kg\,K}}\right] \tag{3.33}$$

where w is the water content within the tissue (given in kg m^{-3}), see table 3.1. A selection of the specific heat capacity and the density of selected materials and organs and components of the human body (and thus of relevance in laser medicine) is listed in table 3.5.

Different relevant parameters can be calculated on the basis of the specific heat capacity and the density. For example, the energy density Q_b required for heating any material such as tissue up to its boiling point is given by

Table 3.5. Specific heat capacity c and density ρ of selected materials and organs and components of the human body [18].

Material/organ/component	Specific heat capacity c in kJ kg^{-1} K^{-1}	Density ρ kg m^{-3}
Copper	0.385	8933
Blood	3.84	900
Water	4.183	1000
Brain	3.6	1040
Liver	3.6	900
Air	1.005	1.290
Skin	3.15	–
Bone	1.3	–
Muscle	3.72	–
Kidney	3.89	–

$$Q_b = \rho c \Delta T. \tag{3.34}$$

Moreover, the energy density required for vaporisation Q_v can be determined according to

$$Q_v = \rho L_v \tag{3.35}$$

where L_v is the so-called latent heat for vaporisation[19]. The volume vaporised by laser irradiation with the laser power P is then given by

$$V = \frac{P}{Q_v + Q_b}. \tag{3.36}$$

It can also be determined considering the focus diameter of the laser beam $2w_0$, the feed speed v,[20] and the cutting depth d_{cut} according to

$$V = 2w_0 \cdot v \cdot d_{cut}. \tag{3.37}$$

Accordingly, the cutting depth is given by

$$d_{cut} = \frac{P}{2w_0 \cdot v(Q_v + Q_b)}. \tag{3.38}$$

Heat conduction

Heat conduction is the movement of heat within a body where the heat transfer is due to collisions of particles. It is thus a transfer of energy, to be precise, the internal energy of a body. Heat transfer always occurs from hotter to colder regions with the temperature T_1 and T_2, respectively. The difference in temperature of these regions $T_1 - T_2$ is described by a temperature gradient which—in the one-dimensional case of an ideal and homogeneous body—is related to the length l and the area A of the volume where heat conduction occurs, as shown schematically in figure 3.25.

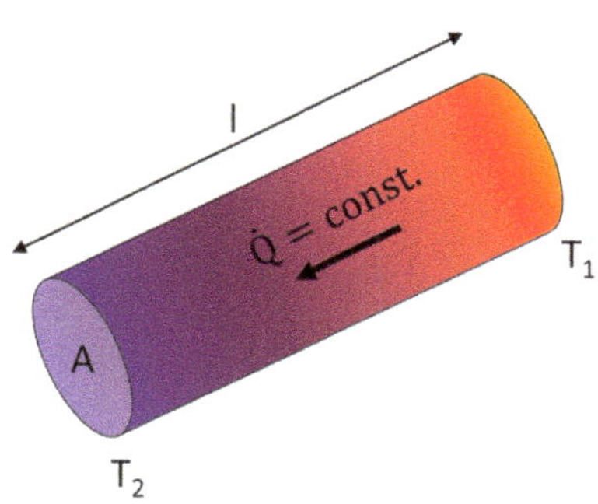

Figure 3.25. Visualisation of heat conduction in a cylindrical body with the base area A and the length l due to a difference in temperature $(T_2 - T_1)$, leading to a constant heat flow $\dot{Q}$.

[19] The latent heat for vaporisation of tissue amounts to $L_V = 2.3 \times 10^6$ J kg^{-1}.

[20] The feed speed is the relative lateral speed between a work piece (e.g. tissue) and a laser beam outlet nozzle.

The heat flow $\Delta Q/\Delta t$ is proportional to the temperature gradient. The conduction of thermal or heat energy ΔQ within a time interval Δt from the hotter to the colder region is then described by the inter-relationship

$$\frac{\Delta Q}{\Delta t} = \lambda \cdot A \frac{T_1 - T_2}{l}. \tag{3.39}$$

The proportionality factor λ is the thermal or heat conductivity, given in W m^{-1} K^{-1}. This constant is generally low for gases, but high for metals. As shown by the comparison listed in table 3.6, it is moderate for human tissue or organs.

One has to consider that in contrast to other material characteristics, the heat conductivity does not significantly depend on temperature. As an example, the heat conductivity of water amounts to 0.62 W m^{-1} K^{-1} at a temperature of 37 °C and to 0.64 W m^{-1} K^{-1} at 57 °C. As listed in table 3.6, tissue exhibits a heat conductivity in the range from 0.3 to 0.5 W m^{-1} K^{-1} where the actual value depends on the particular water content. This is also expressed by the approximation [16, 21]

$$\lambda = \left(0.06 + 0.57\frac{w}{\rho}\right)\left[\frac{\mathrm{W}}{\mathrm{m\,K}}\right]. \tag{3.40}$$

Here, w is the content of water within the tissue and ρ is the density of tissue, compare equation (3.33). When introducing external heat into a body, for example by means of laser irradiation, a phase transition occurs if a critical temperature is exceeded. The heated material is then either molten or vaporised since the bond forces of atoms or molecules cannot withstand the continuously increasing heat conduction. The heat-induced breaking of the internal arrangement of a solid body in the first step or a liquid in the second step thus gives rise to increased entropy[21]. Once the process of phase transition temperature is reached, a further constant heat

Table 3.6. Heat conductivity λ of selected materials and organs and components of the human body [19, 20].

Material/organ/component	Heat conductivity λ in W m^{-1} K^{-1}
Air	0.02
Adipose tissue	≈ 0.3
Aqueous tissue	≈ 0.5
Cartilage (water content = 60–70%)	0.36
Kidney (water content = 84%)	0.55
Liver (water content = 77%)	0.57
Water	0.58
Blood	0.62
Copper	418.00

[21] The entropy is a measure for the disarrangement of a physical system, e.g. a solid or a liquid.

supply does not cause an increase in temperature of the molten or vaporised volume until the phase transition process is terminated.

Heat dissipation by blood flow

The thermal energy introduced by incident laser irradiation is not exclusively diverted from the irradiated zone by heat conduction. Another contributing effect is heat dissipation or convection by the blood flow within the vascular system. This means that blood which exhibits the normal arterial temperature of approximately 37 °C enters the irradiated zone and is instantaneously heated and then further transported by the venous branch of circulation. This system could thus be compared to a technical cooling circuit where the quantity of heat dissipation mainly depends on the specific heat capacity of the blood and its components[22]. The contribution of this mechanism in cooling of tissue and its temperature distribution can be determined on the basis of the so-called perfusion time of the blood t_b, given by

$$t_b = \frac{1}{v_b \cdot \rho} \tag{3.41}$$

with v_b being the blood circulation rate, as listed in table 3.7, and ρ being the density of the irradiated tissue[23]. As visualised in figure 3.26, the perfusion time thus gives the duration of heat transport by blood circulation.

Since different types of tissue exhibit quite different blood circulation rates and densities, the calculation of the perfusion time should be performed for each particular case. It finally indicates the time required for a complete replacement of the blood within a defined volume (i.e. the irradiated one). A significant contribution of heat dissipation by blood flow occurs if the irradiation time is the same order of magnitude or even higher than the perfusion time. This especially applies to laser processes employing continuous wave laser sources where the mechanism of blood

Table 3.7. Blood circulation rate of selected organs and components of the human body [22].

Organ/component	Blood circulation rate in ml min^{-1} g^{-1}
Kidney	3.4
Brain	0.45–1
Tissue	0.15–0.5
Muscles (arms)	0.2–0.07
Adipose tissue	0.012–0.015

[22] As an approximation, the specific heat capacity of water of 4.2 kJ kg^{-1} K^{-1} (at $T = 20$ °C) may be used for calculating heat dissipation by blood flow. However, the specific heat capacity of tissue can reach quite different values in the range 2.1–3.8 kJ kg^{-1} K^{-1}.

[23] The tissue density is found in the range $\rho = 900$–1600 kg m^{-3}.

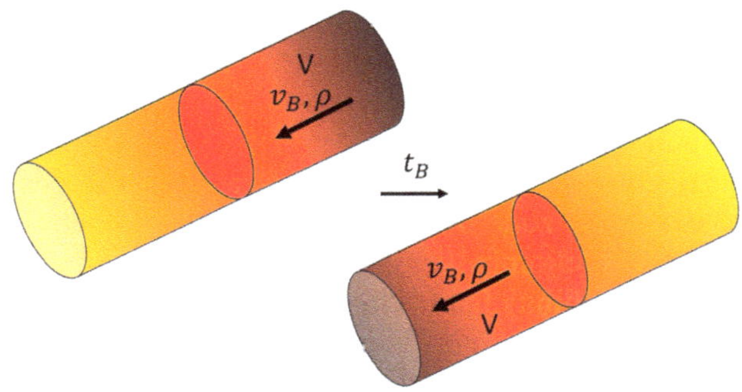

Figure 3.26. Visualisation of the perfusion time t_b, i.e. the duration of heat transport by blood circulation at the blood circulation rate v_b within a certain volume V of tissue with the density ρ.

flow-induced cooling is the dominating convection mechanism which significantly improves heat dissipation. For an irradiated zone without any heat dissipation by blood flow, the decrease in temperature is proportional to the reciprocal of the distance r from the local heat source[24], i.e. the point of incidence of laser irradiation. In contrast, cooling by blood flow introduces an additional term which is described by an exponential decay. The distribution of temperature T is then given by

$$T \propto \frac{1}{r} e^{\left(\frac{-d_{\mathrm{th}}}{r}\right)}. \tag{3.42}$$

Here, d_{th} is the thermal depth of penetration, defined by

$$d_{\mathrm{th}} = \sqrt{\kappa t_{\mathrm{b}}} \tag{3.43}$$

with κ being the thermal diffusivity as described in more detail in section 3.2.2. Notable impact on the blood flow occurs if the dimension of the irradiated zone exceeds the above-defined thermal depth of penetration. In the opposite case, heat dissipation is mainly due to heat diffusion by temperature gradients.

3.2 Interaction of laser irradiation and biological tissue

When irradiated with laser irradiation, a number of quite different effects can arise in biological tissue. These effects are primarily due to the interaction of photons with molecules or molecule assemblies and strongly depend on the application parameters. These include the laser wavelength, its intensity (for continuous wave lasers) or energy density, also known as fluence (for pulsed lasers), and the duration of exposition, i.e. the interaction time. The resulting mechanisms of interaction can be classified into three main categories, (i) photochemical processes, (ii) thermal

[24] Here, the quantity symbol r, i.e., the abbreviation for 'radius', is used for the distance since the profile of an incident laser beam is usually rotational-symmetric, thus inducing a rotational-symmetric local point heat source.

processes, and (iii) nonlinear processes. An overview of such laser–tissue interactions is shown in figure 3.27.

It turns out that photochemical processes occur at low intensities and high interaction times, whereas thermal processes (thermal ablation, vaporisation, and coagulation) are induced at medium intensities and interaction times. Nonlinear effects finally arise in the case of high intensities ($I > 10^7$ W cm^{-2}) and ultra-short interaction times in the nanosecond or picosecond range. Here, the incident laser irradiation causes a modification of the optical properties of tissue and especially its absorbance by the physical effect of multi-photon absorption. This leads to an optical breakdown, i.e. the formation of plasma within the tissue. The plasma then generates an acoustic shock wave which ruptures the tissue mechanically during propagation. This effect is referred to as photo-disruption and is presented in more detail in section 3.2.4.

3.2.1 Photochemical impact on tissue

Incident light can cause a number of different photochemical effects in tissue. For instance, the irradiation of living tissue at low laser power may impact the proliferation of cells. Moreover, several works on the interaction of photons and *in vitro* cell cultures as well as wound healing by means of bio-stimulation have been reported in the past[25]. Intense and controlled clinical investigations have shown that photons are also capable of inducing stimulating effects *in vivo*. The energy of photons can have a notable influence on the cellular metabolism or intracellular

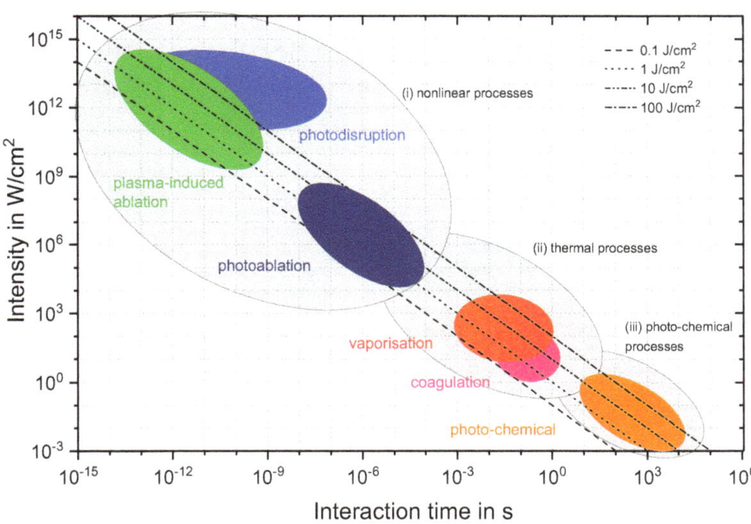

Figure 3.27. Visualisation of laser–tissue interactions dependent on intensity and interaction time (adapted from [23]).

[25] Here, helium neon lasers at a wavelength of $\lambda = 633$ nm or diode lasers ($\lambda = 820$ nm) were applied. It should be noted that some of the reported results are not verified.

signalling cascades when absorbed at suitable structures such as cytochrome-c-oxidase[26] or photoactive porphyrins. This effect is applied for the so-called low level laser therapy (LLLT)[27]. Here, the photons of incident infrared light is absorbed by mitochondria and the inserted energy leads to an increased production of adenosine triphosphate (ATP), reactive oxygen species (ROS), and nitric oxide (NO) within the cell, as shown in figure 3.28.

As a consequence, the cell's energy production is increased, leading to different intermediate steps such as a modulation of the concentration of cytokine and a higher activity of second messengers, for example cyclic adenosine monophosphate (cAMP) or calcium ions (Ca^{2+}). Finally, gene transcription occurs via activation of transcription factors within the cell, giving rise to an increased cell growth, proliferation, and motility [24]. This effect contributes to wound healing, tissue repair and tissue death prevention as well as an increased aeration, i.e. the oxygen enrichment within tissue. In any case, the dose of light must be determined and maintained carefully in order to avoid overdoses. This especially applies for the spectral ranges which are capable of inducing increased activity including the wavelengths 633 nm, 690 nm, and 900 nm as well as the wavelength range 810–820 nm.

3.2.2 Thermal impact on tissue

From a medical point of view, thermal effects of laser irradiation are the coagulation and vaporisation of tissue at comparatively low laser intensity (1–10^6 W cm^{-2}) and high irradiation or interaction time (a number of milliseconds to a number of seconds). The resulting thermal impact can be described on the basis of the laser-induced increase in temperature and the duration of temperature influence.

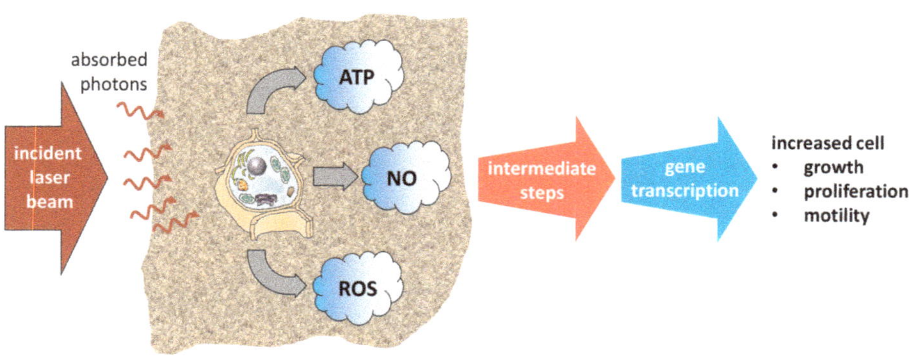

Figure 3.28. Basic mechanisms and cellular signal transduction pathways as induced by low level laser therapy (LLLT) (adapted from [8]).

---

[26] This trans-membrane protein features high absorbance in the near infrared wavelength range.

[27] The abbreviation LLLT is also used for low level light therapy where infrared light emitting diodes or other light sources such as lamps are employed instead of lasers.

Depending on the grade of heating, different tissue degradations and damage result, as shown in figure 3.29.

Thermal damage of tissue, which is basically due to chemical reactions, is generally described by the so-called Arrhenius equation, given by

$$k = A \cdot e^{-\left(\frac{E_a}{k_B \cdot T}\right)}. \tag{3.44}$$

Here, k is the rate constant of a chemical reaction, A is the pre-exponential factor, i.e. a constant for a chemical reaction, E_a is the activation energy required for inducing the chemical reaction, k_B is the Boltzmann constant, and T is the absolute temperature. This equation implies that the damage threshold of tissue depends on (i) the laser power or energy which supplies the activation energy, (ii) temperature, and (iii) the interaction time as considered by the pre-exponential factor, which is also referred to as the frequency factor, given in s^{-1}. The exponential dependence of the temperature on the interaction time, as given by the Arrhenius equation, is shown in figure 3.30.

One has to consider that the thermal impact of incident laser irradiation on any material such as tissue is strongly dependent on the interaction time. Here, a thermal and a quasi-non-thermal regime can be identified. Typical so-called thermal laser-induced effects are coagulation and vaporisation of tissue (and other biological media such as bones). Here, comparatively long interaction times lead to an accumulation of heat within the tissue, consequently resulting in the above-mentioned thermal effects[28]. In contrast, short interaction times give rise to quasi-non-thermal effects such as photo-

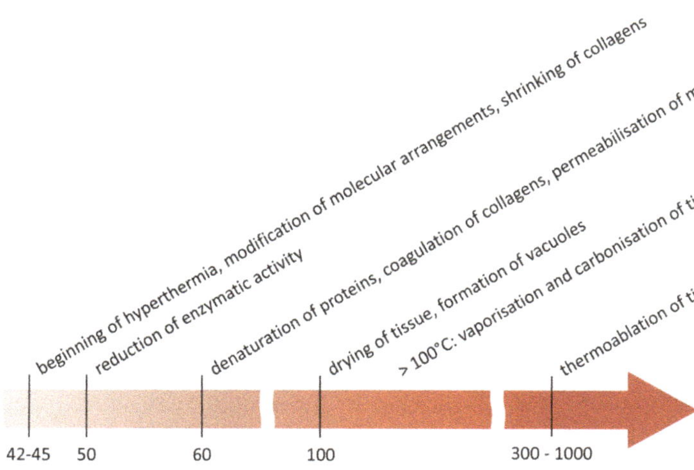

Figure 3.29. Quantitative visualisation of temperature-dependence of different tissue degradations and damage.

[28] It should be noted that the effective interaction time does not only depend on the duration of irradiation, but also on the laser pulse duration and repetition rate of the laser pulses. The heating of any irradiated medium results from these two parameters. Even for short laser pulses in the picosecond range, notable accumulation of heat may occur at high repetition rates.

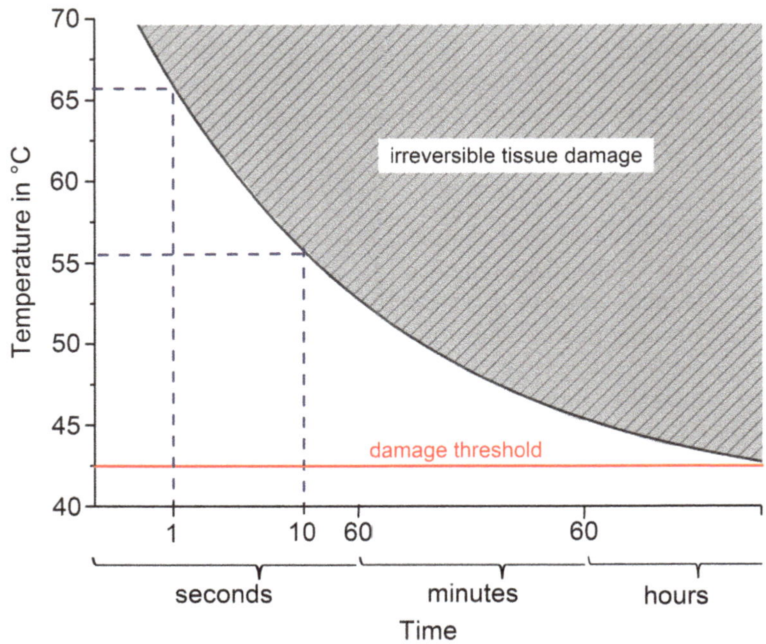

Figure 3.30. Typical time-temperature-dependence of tissue degradation and damage (adapted from [8]).

ablation. This regime is characterised by a negligible heat affected zone (HAZ) around the actual laser-treated area where the size of the acceptable HAZ may significantly differ, depending on the particular application[29]. In the case of tissue, an irreversible effect within the HAZ is coagulation, which is induced by two mechanisms, (i) heating by scattered laser irradiation, see section 3.1.1, and (ii) heat conduction, as described in more detail in section 3.1.3.

When subjected to incident laser irradiation, a certain volume of tissue with the ablation depth x_{abl} is directly heated and ablated if the inserted energy exceeds the ablation threshold. As shown in figure 3.31, a fraction of the laser power or energy is dissipated into non-ablated regions around the actually irradiated area. According to the Beer–Lambert law, laser power or energy is thus absorbed within such regions. Since the energy required for coagulation of tissue is approximately 10% of the energy required for evaporation, the indirectly heated tissue is partially coagulated. As an estimation, the thickness of the coagulated layer roughly corresponds to the optical penetration depth x_{opt} of the incident laser light. It is thus the reciprocal value of the absorption coefficient according to equation (3.13).

Moreover, a certain volume of tissue is further slightly heated by heat conduction, also referred to as thermal diffusion. The depth of thermal diffusion x_{diff} can be calculated on the basis of a one-dimensional model, see section 3.1.2, and is given by

[29] The size of the HAZ plays an essential and important role during laser-assisted *in situ* keratomileusis (LASIK). Here, very small HAZ in the range of some micrometres or even smaller are required, whereas a HAZ of some hundreds of micrometres may be acceptable during laser cutting of bones.

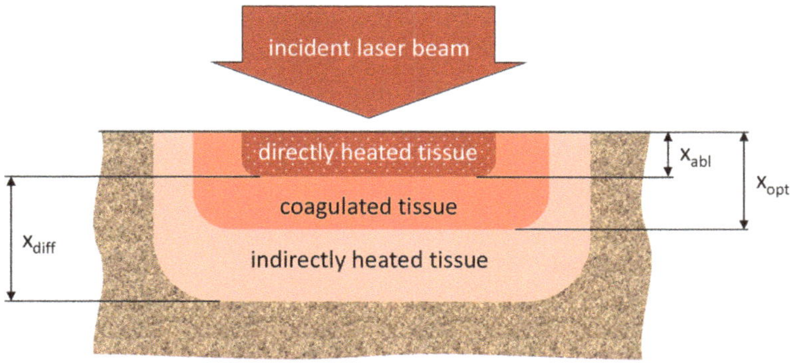

Figure 3.31. Comparison of ablation depth x_{abl}, the optical penetration depth x_{opt}, and the depth of thermal diffusion x_{diff}.

$$x_{\mathrm{diff}} = \sqrt{2 \cdot \frac{\lambda}{\rho \cdot c} \cdot t}. \tag{3.45}$$

Here, λ is the thermal conductivity, ρ is the density, c is the specific heat capacity, and t is time, i.e. the interaction time as given by the duration of laser irradiation. The expression $\lambda/\rho \cdot c$ is also referred to as the thermal diffusivity κ (given in $\mathrm{m}^2\,\mathrm{s}^{-1}$). On the basis of equation (3.45), the diffusion time t_{diff} can be defined. At this point in time, the optical penetration depth corresponds to the range of heat diffusion[30]. It is given by

$$t_{\mathrm{diff}} = \frac{x_{\mathrm{opt}}^2}{\kappa} \tag{3.46}$$

The diffusion time allows estimating the size of the laser-induced heat affected zone qualitatively on the basis of the interaction time t: For $t < t_{\mathrm{diff}}$, the heat affected zone, i.e. the coagulated zone, corresponds to the optical penetration depth. In the case of $t > t_{\mathrm{diff}}$, the coagulated zone is increased due to heat conduction.

In practice, the interaction time t is given by the laser pulse duration τ_{p}. For laser pulse durations shorter than the diffusion time, the interaction is subject to thermal confinement. This means that the pulse energy is converted into heat within a volume of tissue V_{tissue} given by

$$V_{\mathrm{tissue}} = \frac{w_0^2 \cdot \pi}{\mu_{\mathrm{a}}} = w_0^2 \cdot \pi \cdot x_{\mathrm{opt}}. \tag{3.47}$$

This volume thus follows from the diameter $2w_0$ of the incident laser beam and the absorption coefficient μ_{a} and the optical penetration depth x_{opt}, respectively. Thermal confinement occurs if the ratio of the laser pulse duration and the diffusion

[30] For instance, the diffusion time amounts to approximately 1 ms for CO_2 laser irradiation (wavelength $\lambda = 10.6\ \mu\mathrm{m}$) within tissue with an absorption coefficient of $\mu_{\mathrm{a}} = 500\ \mathrm{cm}^{-1}$.

time is equal to or lower than one. This condition is typically described by the non-dimensional characteristic diffusion time t^*_{diff} according to

$$t^*_{\text{diff}} = \frac{\tau_{\text{p}}}{t_{\text{diff}}} \leqslant 1. \tag{3.48}$$

3.2.3 Photo-ablation of tissue

In contrast to thermal ablation, photo-ablation of tissue stands out due to a reduction in thermal effects and the HAZ, respectively. This mechanism occurs at high laser intensity and low interaction time and short laser pulse duration, respectively, as shown in figure 3.22. The approach of applying short-term and high-intensity laser irradiation gives rise to a rapid heating of tissue and the formation of thermo-elastic tension which contributes to material removal. The amount and temporal behaviour of such tension is generally described by the sound velocity c_{a} within a medium, the laser pulse duration τ_{p}, the optical penetration depth $x_{\text{opt}} = 1/\mu_{\text{a}}$, and the so-called Grüneisen coefficient Γ. This coefficient is a thermo-physical parameter, given by

$$\Gamma = \left(\frac{\partial \sigma}{\partial E}\right)_V = \frac{\alpha}{\rho c_v \kappa_T}. \tag{3.49}$$

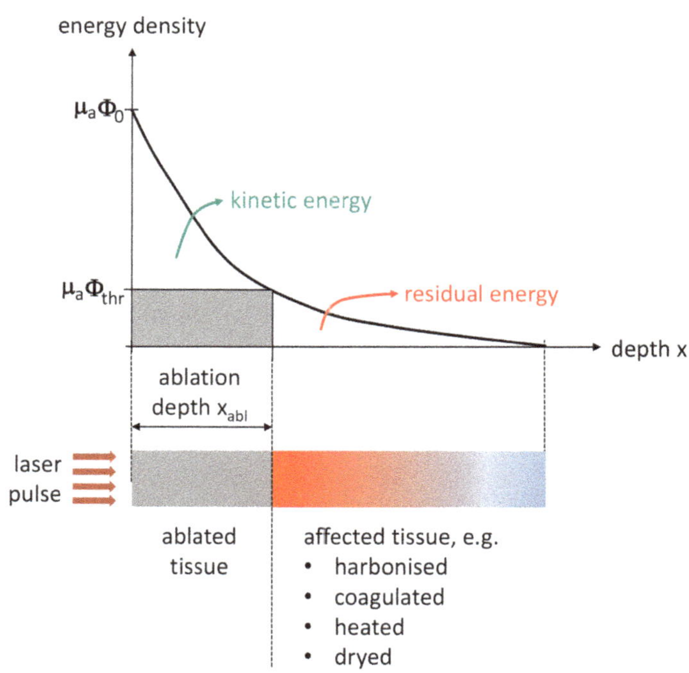

Figure 3.32. Schematic of the blow-off model (adapted from [25]).

Here, α is the coefficient of thermal expansion, ρ is the density, c_v the specific heat capacity of a constant volume, and κ_T is the isothermal compressibility[31]. Comparable to thermal confinement as described in the previous section, the so-called stress confinement can be defined. Here, the tissue is heated extremely rapidly and the laser pulse duration is shorter than the expansion time of the thermo-elastic stress wave t_{stress} within the heated volume, given by

$$t_{\mathrm{stress}} = \frac{1}{c_{\mathrm{a}}\mu_{\mathrm{a}}}. \tag{3.50}$$

During laser irradiation, stress confinement dominates if the non-dimensional characteristic expansion time of the thermo-elastic stress wave t^*_{stress} is equal to or lower than one:

$$t^*_{\mathrm{stress}} = \frac{\tau_{\mathrm{p}}}{t_{\mathrm{stress}}} \leqslant 1. \tag{3.51}$$

In this case, the laser-induced stress wave leads to an (mainly mechanical) ejection of tissue material. In the case of dominating thermal confinement, material removal is described by the so-called blow-off model, shown schematically in figure 3.32. This model allows the calculation of the ablation depth during photo-ablation [25].

For initiating any laser ablation process, a certain threshold energy density, also known as threshold fluence Φ_{thr}, given by

$$\Phi_{\mathrm{thr}}(\delta) = \Phi_0 \cdot e^{-[\mu_{\mathrm{a}} \cdot x_{\mathrm{abl}}]} \tag{3.52}$$

has to be exceeded. Here, Φ_0 is the maximum fluence. Once the ablation process has started, the ablation depth x_{abl} then increases until a certain saturation value is reached. The threshold fluence is directly related to the threshold energy Q_{thr} which is required for abrupt vaporisation of tissue by short-term heating. The energy dQ absorbed within a tissue layer with the thickness dz is given by

$$dQ = \mu_{\mathrm{a}} Q_{\mathrm{thr}} dz. \tag{3.53}$$

Relating to an ablation process, the minimum energy dQ which is required for heating an infinitely thin layer with the thickness dz from its initial temperature T_0 to the boiling temperature T_{b}, corresponding to a change in temperature ΔT, follows from

$$dQ = \rho(c_{\mathrm{w}}\Delta T + L_{\mathrm{v}})A dz. \tag{3.54}$$

Here, ρ is the density of the material and L_{v} the latent heat of vaporisation[32]. Disregarding losses of energy which may for example occur due to heat conduction, the required threshold energy thus amounts to

[31] The isothermal compressibility is a measure used in thermodynamics and fluid mechanics. It indicates the relative volume change of a medium induced by a change in pressure and is thus also given by the reciprocal value of the bulk modulus of elasticity E.

[32] For instance, the latent heat of vaporisation of water amounts to $L_{\mathrm{v}} = 2.3 \cdot 10^3$ kJ kg^{-1}.

$$Q_{\text{thr}} = \frac{\rho(c_{\text{w}}\Delta T + L_{\text{v}})A}{\mu_{\text{a}}}. \tag{3.55}$$

The threshold fluence[33] is then given by

$$\Phi_{\text{thr}} = \frac{\rho(c_{\text{w}}\Delta T + L_{\text{v}})}{\mu_{\text{a}}}. \tag{3.56}$$

Based on this parameter and considering the absorption coefficient μ_{a} additionally, the ablation depth can be determined according to

$$x_{\text{abl}} = \frac{1}{\mu_{\text{a}}} \ln\left(\frac{\Phi_0}{\Phi_{\text{thr}}}\right). \tag{3.57}$$

The impact of the absorption coefficient on the ablation process, i.e. the dependence of the ablation depth on the laser fluence is shown by the examples in figures 3.33 and 3.34.

Finally, an overview on the presented laser–tissue interaction's thermal confinement and stress confinement (and no confinement additionally) is given in figure 3.35. Here the optical penetration depth is plotted versus the typical pulse duration of the particular laser source mentioned. It turns out that the mechanism of stress confinement is dominating in the case of short-pulse lasers, whereas the application

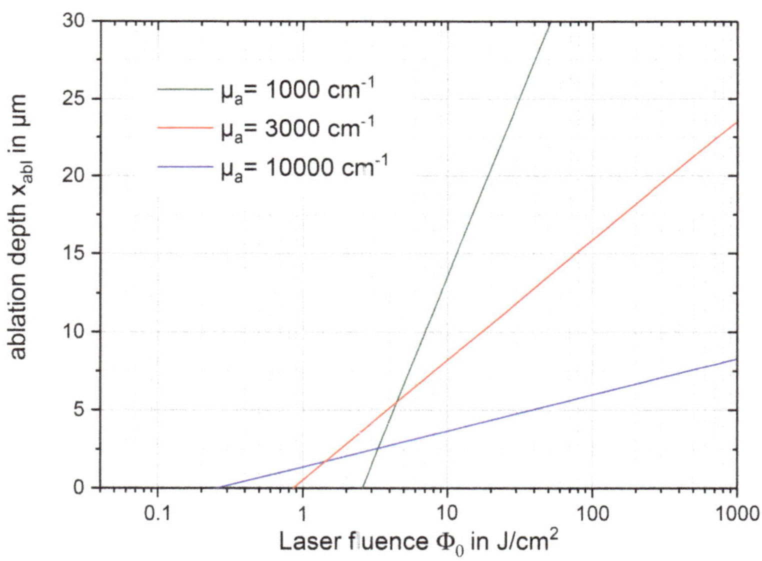

Figure 3.33. Ablation depth versus laser fluence for three different media with different absorption coefficients μ_{a}.

[33] In the case of water, the threshold fluence amounts to $\Phi_{\text{thr}} = 2580/\mu_{\text{a}}$ mJ mm^{-2} when assuming heating from the mean body temperature $T_0 = 37$ °C to a final temperature of $T = 100$ °C and taking a constant and linear absorption coefficient as a basis.

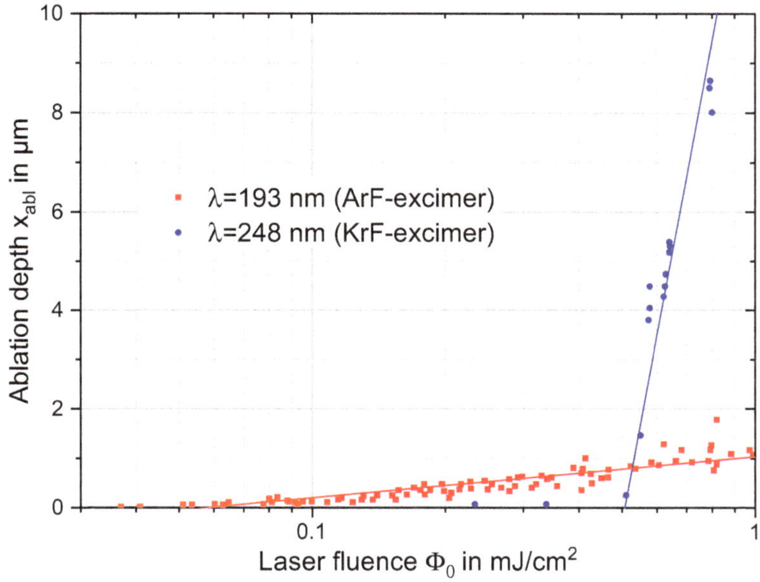

Figure 3.34. Ablation depth versus laser fluence of callused skin for two different laser wavelengths (data taken from [26, 27]).

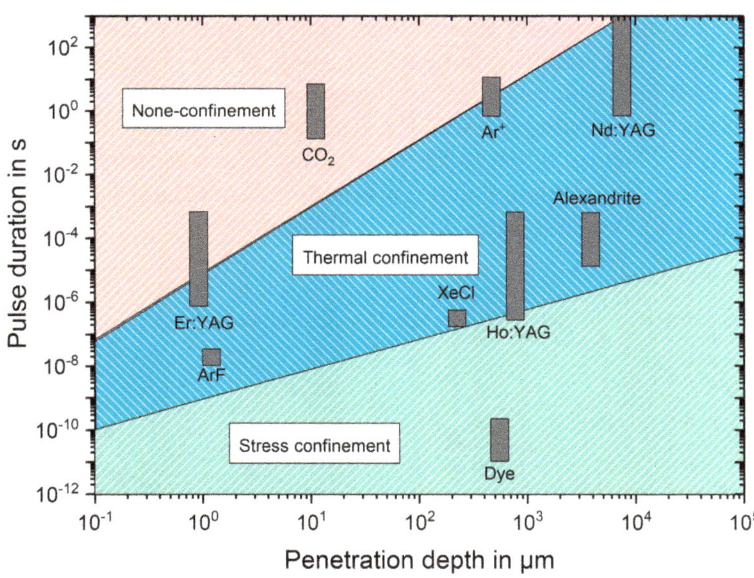

Figure 3.35. Optical penetration depth versus typical pulse duration of laser sources used in medicine (adapted from [8]).

of longer pulses gives rise to thermal confinement. For extremely long laser pulses, no confinement but pure heating occurs.

3.2.4 Photo-disruption and plasma-induced ablation of tissue

The intensity of focussed laser irradiation with pulse durations in the nanosecond, picosecond or femtosecond range amounts to an average value of approximately $I = 10^{12}$ W cm^{-2} and may reach even higher values, depending on the pulse duration. This means that electric fields with extremely high electric field strengths are found in such laser foci. As a consequence, electrons can be torn out of atoms and an optical breakdown can be induced. An optical breakdown comes along with the formation of a plasma and an acoustic shock wave which is finally capable of disrupting tissue mechanically. This effect is referred to as photo-disruption. When exceeding an intensity of approximately 10^{11} W cm^{-2}, nonlinear absorption of light occurs. In this case, multi-photon absorption causes the ionisation of atoms and the accompanying formation of plasma. This effect is strongly intensity-dependent; multi-photon absorption scales with the fourth power of intensity. The free electrons generated in the course of the process are accelerated by inverse bremsstrahlung in the electromagnetic field of the focussed laser irradiation and contribute to the generation of further free electrons by collision ionisation. As shown in figure 3.36, this leads to an avalanche effect where the number of electrons is doubled by each collision.

The electrons exhibit very high velocities and energies, respectively. Further, such laser-induced plasmas typically lead to high local pressures in the range 20–60 bar. As a consequence, a cavitation bubble consisting of water vapour is formed. In addition, laser-induced plasmas feature high electron densities (10^{15}–10^{17} cm^{-3}). This gives rise to an increased absorbance; incident laser light is efficiently absorbed within the plasma. Hence, tissue can be ablated at laser wavelengths which are not absorbed by tissue in its original state, a mixture of solid and liquid components. This approach is known as plasma-induced ablation.

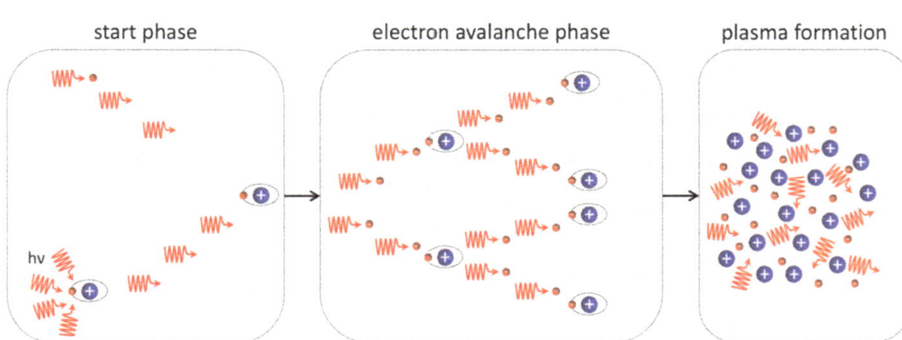

Figure 3.36. Different phases of the plasma formation process as induced by ultra-short laser pulses with high intensity.

3.3 Tissue optics and laser–tissue interactions—the bottom line

- Biological tissue is a complex and optically inhomogeneous medium.
- All physical mechanisms and influencing parameters related to the propagation of light have to be considered for the entire description of the optical properties of tissue.
- Relevant optical properties of tissue are refraction, reflection, absorption and scattering; all these parameters are wavelength-dependent.
- Refraction is defined as the change of propagation direction of light at interfaces of media with different indices of refraction.
- The angle of refraction follows from the indices of refraction of the involved media and the angle of incidence of light, as described by Snell's law.
- Reflection generally occurs at any interface of media with different indices of refraction.
- The amount of reflection, i.e. the reflectance, results from the difference in index of refraction of the involved optical media, the angle of incidence and the polarisation of light, as described by the Fresnel equations.
- From an energetic point of view, absorption is the conversion of incident light energy into another form of energy, normally heat.
- When passing an optical medium, intensity of incident light is successively reduced, as described by the Beer–Lambert law, where absorption is represented by the medium's absorption coefficient.
- The reciprocal value of the absorption coefficient gives the optical depth of penetration.
- Scattering occurs at the smallest particles within an optical medium and could be described as diffuse reflection resulting in complex optical paths.
- Each scattering object, also referred to as a scatter centre, exhibits a scattering cross section.
- There are two different main types of scattering, Rayleigh scattering and Mie scattering. The type of scattering follows from the size of the scatter centre with respect to the wavelength of incident and interacting light.
- The angular distribution of scattered light indicates the change in propagation direction of all involved photons.
- The predominance of backscattering, isotropic scattering or forward-scattering can be described by the so-called anisotropy factor.
- Due to the number of interacting mechanisms, modelling the distribution of light in biological tissue is a complex task where three approaches, modelling by the Beer–Lambert law, modelling by the diffusion approximation, or Monte Carlo simulations are applied.
- The conversion of laser light energy into heat is directly related to the thermal properties of tissue, heat storage, heat conduction and heat dissipation.
- Generally, heat storage is a medium's capability for accumulating heat, leading to an increase in temperature. It is mainly described by the density and the specific heat capacity of a medium.

- Heat conduction leads to the cooling of a heated medium due to a temperature gradient and is described by heat conductivity. In biological tissue, such cooling is further supported by heat dissipation by blood flow.
- Incident laser light can give rise to different effects on tissue such as for example photochemical and thermal impact.
- The main thermal impacts of laser light on tissue are drying, coagulation, carbonisation and vaporisation.
- If induced by laser irradiation, removal of material is referred to as ablation; there are two different main types of ablation mechanisms, thermal ablation and photo-ablation.
- Laser-induced removal of tissue can also be achieved by photodissruption or plasma-induced ablation at high laser pulse energies.

References

[1] Berlien H P and Müller G 2000 *Angewandte Lasermedizin—Lehr und Handbuch für Praxis und Klinik* 3rd edn (Berlin: Laser- und Medizin-Technologie) ISBN 3-609-70510-8
[2] Rowe D J, Smith D and Wilkinson J S 2017 *Sci. Rep.* **7** 7356
[3] Giannios P, Toutouzas K G, Matiatou M, Stasinos K, Konstadoulakis M M, Zografos G C and Moutzouris K 2016 *Sci. Rep.* **6** 27910
[4] Hale G M and Querry M R 1973 *Appl. Opt.* **12** 555–63
[5] Marwitz H 1990 *Praxis der Holografie: Grundlagen, Standard-und Spezialverfahren* (Germany: Expert-Verlag)
[6] Gerhard C 2016 *Tutorium Optik: Ein verständlicher Überblick für Physiker, Ingenieure und Techniker* (Berlin Heidelberg: Springer)
[7] Kou L, Labrie D and Chylek P 1993 *Appl. Opt.* **32** 3531–40
[8] Christian R and Syrus K 2013 *Lasertherapie der Haut* vol 1 ed R Christian and K Syrus ISBN 978-3-642-29910-0
[9] Cheong W F, Prahl S A and Welch A J 1990 *IEEE J. Quantum Electron.* **26** 2166–85
[10] Ritz J P, Roggan A, Isbert C, Müller G, Buhr H J and Germer C T 2001 *Lasers Surg. Med.* **29** 205–12
[11] Roggan A, Dorschel K, Minet O, Wolff D and Muller G 1995 The optical properties of biological tissue in the near infrared wavelength range *SPIE Press* pp 10–44
[12] Esterowitz L, Hoffman C, Tran D, Levin K, Storm M, Bonner R, Smith P and Leon M 1986 *Proc. SPIE* **605** 32–7
[13] Anderson R R and Parrish J A 1981 *J. Invest. Dermatol.* **77** 13–9
[14] Roggan A 1997 *Dosimetrie thermischer Laseranwendungen in der Medizin: Untersuchung der optischen Gewebeeigenschaften und physikalisch-mathematische Modellentwicklung* (Germany: Ecomed)
[15] Niemz M H 2013 *Laser-issue Interactions: Fundamentals and Applications* (Springer Science & Business Media)
[16] Welch A 1984 *IEEE J. Quantum Electron.* **20** 1471–81
[17] Svaasand L O 1989 *Proc. SPIE* **10305** 103050B
[18] Duck F A 1990 *Physical properties of Tissue—A comprehensive reference book* (New York: Academic)
[19] Weast R C 1982 *CRC Handbook of Chamistry and Physics: A Ready Reference Book of Chemical and Physical Data* (Chemical Rubber)

[20] Svaasand L O 1982 *Med. Phys.* **9** 711–4

[21] Takata A N and Zaneveld L R W 1977 *Laser-induced thermal damage of skin, Tech. rep.* (USAF School Aerospace Medicine)

[22] Svaasand L O, Boerslid T and Oeveraasen M 1985 *Lasers Surg. Med.* **5** 589–602

[23] Boulnois J L 1986 *Lasers Med. Sci.* **1** 47–66

[24] Gao X and Xing D 2009 *J. Biomed. Sci.* **16** 4

[25] Vogel A and Venugopalan V 2003 *Chem. Rev.* **103** 577–644

[26] Pettit G and Ediger M 1996 *Appl. Opt.* **35** 3386–91

[27] Loertscher H, Mandelbaum S, Parrish R K and Parel J M 1986 *Am. J. Ophthalmol.* **102** 217–21

IOP Publishing

Lasers in Medical Diagnosis and Therapy
Basics, applications and future prospects
Stephan Wieneke and Christoph Gerhard

Chapter 4

Lasers in medical diagnosis

In this Chapter a selection of established and novel laser-based diagnosis methods is presented. This includes spectroscopic and microscopic measurement techniques for analytical tasks, wave front sensing for the detection of defective vision, optical coherence tomography for measuring alterations of tissue, and pulse oximetry for the control of the blood flow and oxygen saturation. Moreover, the method of synthetic aperture linking for the detection of rheumatism, optical capnography for monitoring anaesthesia, photoactivation of hematoporphyrin derivative for the diagnosis and treatment of tumours, flow cytometry for the differentiation of cells, and laser-induced fluorescence for early recognition of caries are introduced.

4.1 Spectroscopic measurement techniques

4.1.1 Excitation spectroscopy

The principle of excitation spectroscopy is the indirect measurement of discrete absorption bands via the detection of laser-induced fluorescence which corresponds to these absorption bands. This means that the laser irradiation applied for the measurement is adapted to the absorbing transition from a certain lower energy level (E_i) to a higher one (E_k). Hence, the laser irradiation acts as pump energy. The result of the subsequent spontaneous emission of light is thus directly related to the wavelength and energy, respectively, of the incident, pumping laser irradiation. The number of incident photons n_a which are absorbed can be derived from the interrelationship

$$n_a = N_i n_L \sigma_{ik} \Delta x. \tag{4.1}$$

Here, N_i is the density of the absorbing molecules or atoms, n_L is the total number of incident photons, σ_{ik} is the absorption cross section of the transition from the energy level E_i to the energy level E_k, and Δx is the distance which is covered by the incident

doi:10.1088/978-0-7503-1275-2ch4

laser irradiation. Moreover, the number of photons emitted due to fluorescence n_{FL} is directly related to the number of excited molecules or atoms[1] N_k and the Einstein coefficient[2] for this state A_k according to

$$n_{FL} = N_K A_k. \tag{4.2}$$

The relation of spontaneous and total transition probability is referred to as the quantum efficiency η_k. For $\eta_k = 1$, no radiationless de-excitation of the state E_k occurs and each incident laser photon generates a fluorescence photon ($n_{FL} = n_a$) which represents the most efficient case. The laser-irradiated zone, i.e. the excitation volume, can be described as a point light source; fluorescence photons are thus spherically emitted. As a result, only a moderate fractional amount δ of all generated fluorescence photons is detected in one, angular limited direction via the used photomultipliers with the quantum efficiency η_{PM}. In this case, the number of detected photons n_{ph} is given by

$$n_{ph} = n_a \eta_k \eta_{PM} \delta = N_i n_L \sigma_{ik} \Delta x \eta_k \eta_{PM} \delta. \tag{4.3}$$

The quantum efficiency of modern photomultipliers is approximately 20% and the use of sophisticated optical measurement setups allows the detection of up to 70% of the emitted fluorescence photons. Here, the photons are collected via concentrating reflectors and—as the case may be—additional fibre coupling or optical imaging systems, as shown in figure 4.1.

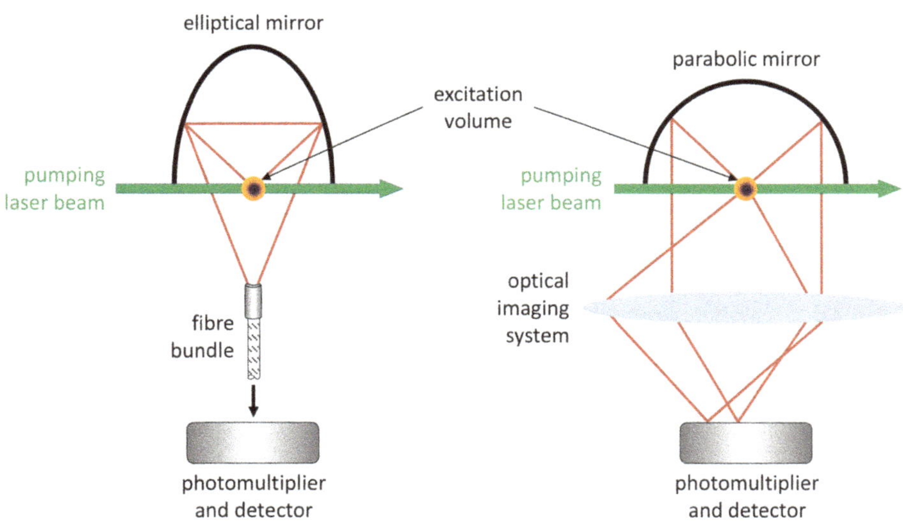

Figure 4.1. Examples for measurement setups for excitation spectroscopy which allow the efficient collection of fluorescence photons by a combination of an elliptical mirror and a fibre bundle (left) or a parabolic mirror and an optical imaging system (right).

[1] I.e. molecules or atoms with electrons which are pumped from the energy level i to the energy level k.

[2] The Einstein coefficient A indicates the probability of the spontaneous emission of light. (In contrast, the probability of the stimulated emission of light for the generation of laser light is quantified by the Einstein coefficient B.)

4.1.2 Infrared spectroscopy

Infrared spectroscopy is a method of molecular spectroscopy. It is based on the use of light in the near and far infrared wavelength range from approximately 800 nm to 1 mm. This allows the identification and quantitative detection of molecules by light-induced excitation of different energy states of molecules such as, for example, vibration. In this case, each vibrational state exhibits its proper energy and frequency[3], respectively. By comparing a measured spectrum to reference databases, the molecular composition of any sample material can thus be determined qualitatively and quantitatively. In practice, an infrared spectrum plots the measured intensity over the so-called wavenumber $\bar{\nu}$, i.e. the reciprocal value of the wavelength λ:

$$\bar{\nu} = \frac{1}{\lambda}. \tag{4.4}$$

The wavenumber is typically given in cm^{-1}. An overview of the wavelength sub-ranges relevant for infrared spectroscopy and the corresponding wavenumbers is given in table 4.1. As shown in figure 4.2, the interaction of infrared light and matter can be classified into three essential mechanisms: first, harmonics of the mid infrared range[4] as well as combination vibrations of molecules are mainly excited in the near infrared wavelength range. Second, vibrations of covalent bonded electrons of molecules (and atoms) occur in the upper, near and mid infrared range. Third, general molecular vibrations are found in the far infrared wavelength range. Such general vibrations are the possible vibrational modes of a molecule, i.e. symmetrical and asymmetrical stretching, bending (sometimes also referred to as scissoring), rocking, wagging, and twisting. Figure 4.3 visualises a selection of general vibrations of carbon dioxide and water.

Due to this wide range of detectable mechanisms and molecular states, respectively, and the accompanying easy and distinct identification and quantification of molecules, infrared spectroscopy is a powerful tool in biotechnology. For instance, mid infrared spectroscopy allows the chemical analysis of organic substances or the determination of the composition of unknown biological samples. Moreover, fast

Table 4.1. Overview of the wavelength sub-ranges of relevance for infrared spectroscopy including the corresponding wavenumber's wavelength sub-range, wavelength in μm, wavenumber in cm^{-1}.

Wavelength sub-range	Wavelength in μm	Wavenumber in cm^{-1}
Near infrared, NIR	0.8–2.5	12 500–4000
Mid infrared, MIR	2.5–25	4000–400
Far infrared, FIR	25–1000	400–10

[3] Typical frequencies of molecular vibrations are found in the range of approximately 10^{13}–10^{14} Hz.
[4] This especially applies for CH-, OH-, and NH-bonds.

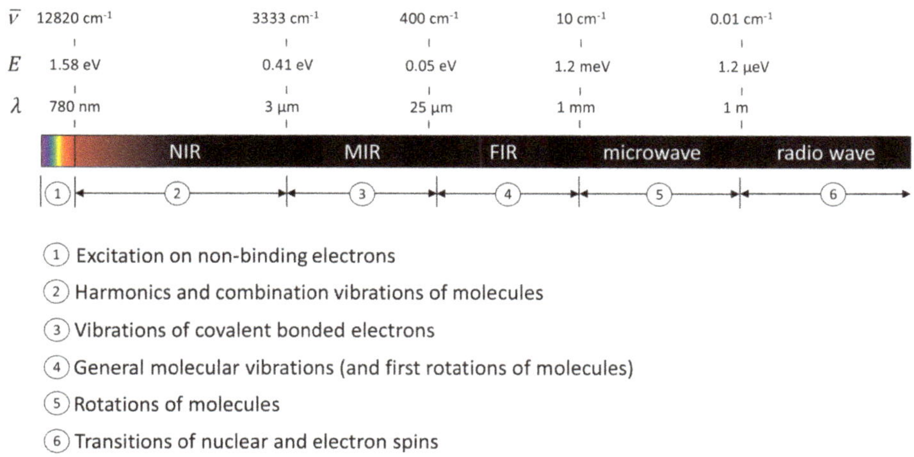

Figure 4.2. Overview on the infrared wavelength range including the particular wavelengths λ and corresponding photon energies E and wavenumbers $\bar{\nu}$ as well as the main mechanisms of interaction in the sub-ranges of the infrared spectrum.

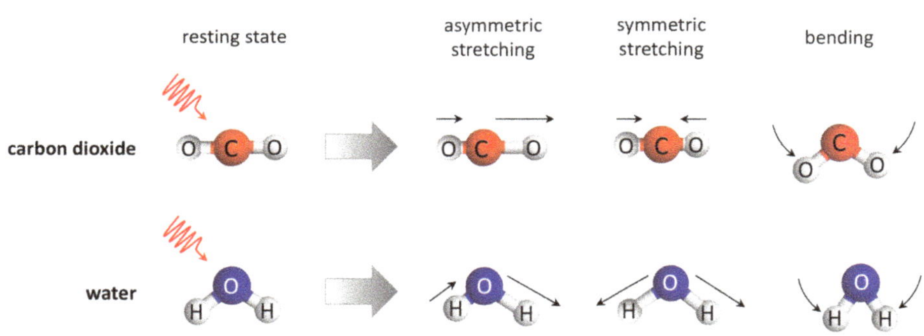

Figure 4.3. Visualisation of different types of molecule vibrations induced by incident infrared light; asymmetric and symmetric stretching as well as bending of carbon dioxide (top) and water (bottom) molecules.

analysis on the basis of computer-assisted evaluation techniques and sufficient reference standards can be performed via near infrared spectroscopy. For the visualisation of the measured spectrum, both absorption and transmission can be displayed principally. However, the evaluation of the infrared absorption characteristic is usually performed by measuring a sample's transmission[5]. This allows fast identification of absorption bands which appear as discrete notches in a transmission spectrum. Such notches are formed due to the fact that specific frequency ranges or discrete frequencies of electromagnetic waves are absorbed by a substance when irradiated.

The absorbed light in the infrared wavelength range is the driving force for the excitation of vibrations and rotations of small molecules or molecule assemblies.

[5] The evaluation of absorption spectra is applied in some special approaches such as for example the so-called attenuated total reflection (ATR) infrared spectroscopy.

Hence, a molecule can clearly be identified on the basis of the absorbed light which, from an energetic point of view, corresponds to the energy required for initiating vibration or rotation. For this purpose, the molecule must exhibit an infrared-active dipole moment[6]. This means that the vibrations must be asymmetric with respect to the symmetry centre of the molecule[7]. However, the absorption bands of some molecules or bonds may not become visible in an infrared spectrum. This can be due to different reasons: (i) the vibration may not be infrared-active, (ii) the absorption band may be weak and stronger bands may superimpose this band of interest, (iii) the superposition of several, closely neighbouring absorption bands may impede or even prevent the identification of a specific absorption band, and finally, (iv) the absorption band may simply be outside the measured spectral range.

Applications of infrared spectroscopy in medicine:

- Examination of humours such as urine, saliva, synovial fluid or blood plasma for the determination of the concentration of essential substances, for example, dextrose, cholesterol, triglyceride, urea, protein, phosphate etc
- Investigation of the structure and interactions of proteins, lipids, carbohydrate and nucleic acids
- Quantitative determination of the composition of tissue samples for clinical examinations and the detection of diseases such as arthritis, multiple sclerosis, Alzheimer's disease and different types of cancer
- Pathological examination for the classification of tissue types without any tracer dyes as usually required for classical histology or fluorescence microscopy
- Different uses in non-invasive diagnosis, e.g. for the measurement of blood glucose.

Basic setup of classical infrared spectrometers

To record the spectrum of polychromatic light its single spectral fractions have to be isolated. This means that every single wavelength which is found within the measured spectrum needs to be measured regarding its intensity. The monochromators required for this task can be realised by different technical approaches. First, so-called non-dispersive apparatus can be used. In this type of spectrometer the isolation of each wavelength is performed by the use of different colour filters; incoming light passes the filters and the final spectrum is reconstructed on the basis of the measured light intensity per filter or wavelength, respectively. This approach features poor spectral resolution and is thus used for some applications where high spectral resolution is not required.

A high resolution can be achieved by so-called dispersive setups, based on optical gratings or prisms, as shown in figure 4.4. Spectral separation of polychromatic light by optical gratings is based on the effect of diffraction and subsequent interference. In contrast, the wavelength-dependence of the index of

[6] The dipole moment can be either an existing one, an alterable one or an inducible one.

[7] Molecules with symmetric vibrations (with respect to the molecule's symmetry centre) are not infrared-active since in the case of such vibration, the dipole moment of the molecule is not altered.

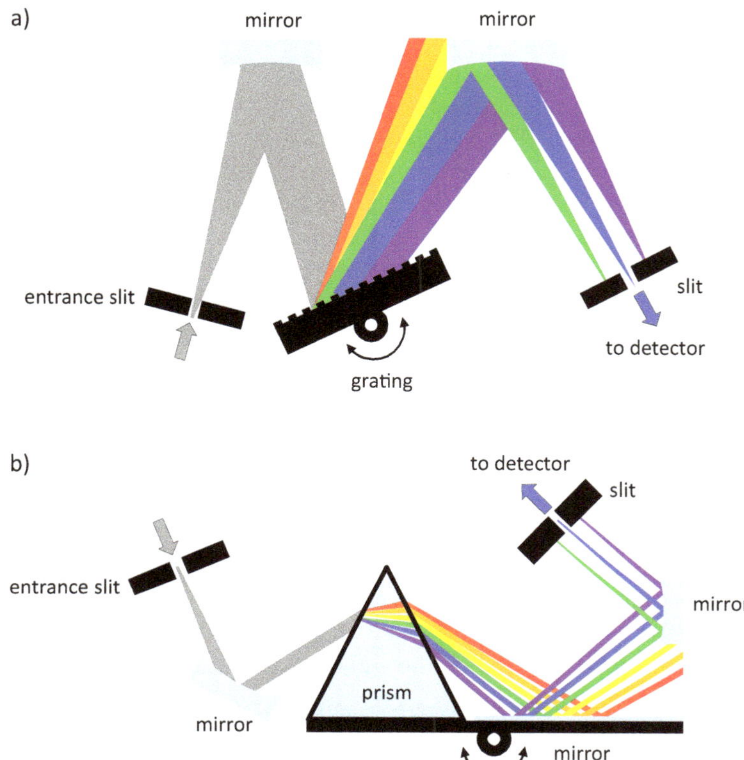

Figure 4.4. Two different types of spectrometers; grating-based Czerny–Turner setup (a) and prism-based setup according to Wadshorth (b) (adapted from [1]).

refraction of optical glasses represents the underlying mechanism for spectral separation by a prism. Even though the latter type is the classical one, modern monochromators or spectrometers are mainly based on gratings. This is due to the fact that the spectral resolution or spectral resolving power *RP*, i.e. the capability of resolving two close wavelengths λ_1 and λ_2, of gratings is much better in comparison to prisms. For instance, the use of blazed gratings which are optimized for a certain diffraction order allows a spectral resolution of 10^4 to be obtained. This means that depending on the particular wavelength range observed, two wavelengths with a spectral distance of just some tens of picometres can be identified and measured separately. Such powerful spectrometers are referred to as echelle spectrometers.

Fourier-transform infrared spectroscopy

A special type of infrared spectrometer is the Fourier-transform infrared (FTIR) spectrometer. Here, the detection of the spectrum is not performed by the use of dispersive elements for successive observation and measurement of single wavelengths, as described in section 4.1.2. The spectrum is instead calculated by a Fourier transform[8] of a measured interferogram. As shown in figure 4.5, the key element of an FTIR spectrometer is thus an interferometer, i.e. a Michelson interferometer (compare figure 4.17) in the present case [2].

Here, a light beam which is emitted by a light source is split into two fractions by a beam splitter. The size of the light source can be altered by a set of different pinholes, placed in a rotatable pinhole wheel, in order to improve the spectral resolution of the setup. The two single light rays produced by the beam splitter are reflected by two mirrors, a fixed one and a movable one. The latter mirror is then moved with respect to the fixed one in order to alter the distance between both mirrors which is measured with the use of an additional pilot laser, see figure 4.5. After reflection at the mirrors, the two light rays then pass the beam splitter and thus interfere with each other. The resulting interferogram contains information on the light frequencies and wavelengths, respectively, and features a maximum, also known as centre burst, at that position where both mirrors featured the same distance, i.e. optical path length, to the beam splitter. For other positions, gently dipping wings are formed around the centre burst. This measured interferogram is finally converted into a spectrum, as shown in figure 4.6 by a Fourier transform.

In comparison to dispersive spectrometer setups, FTIR spectrometers stand out due to short testing times and the accompanying increased signal-to-noise ratio. This allows the detection of weak bands which might be impossible to measure when using a dispersive setup. Moreover, the light efficiency of FTIR spectrometers is

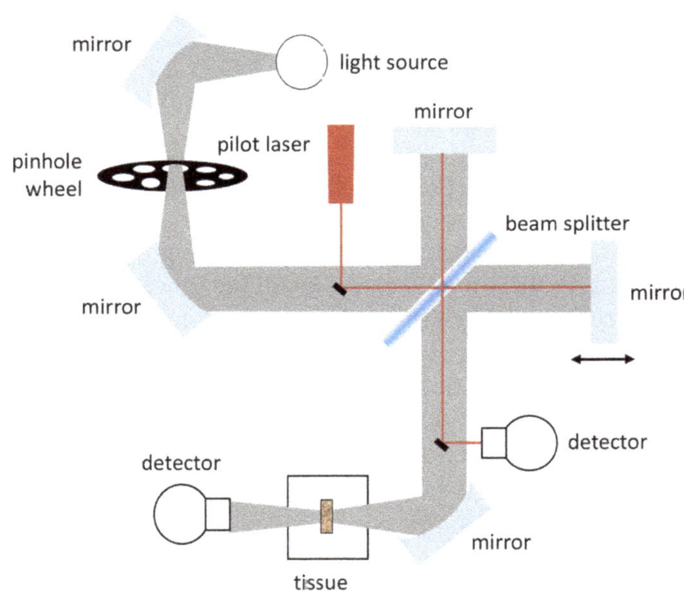

Figure 4.5. Schematic of an FTIR spectrometer setup.

[8] The Fourier transform is a mathematical operation which allows decomposing a time-dependent function into the frequencies (or wavelengths, respectively) which form this function.

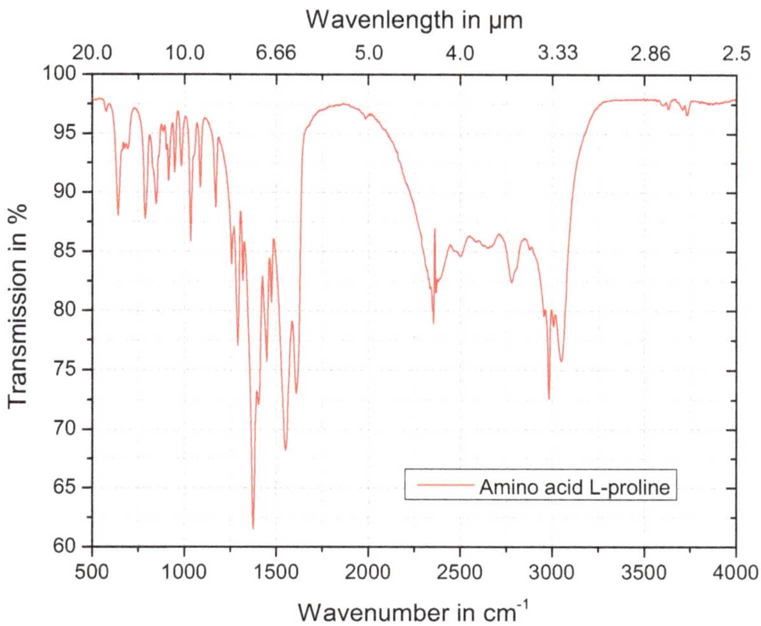

Figure 4.6. FTIR spectrum of amino acid L-proline. (Measured values provided by Anna Scheglov, internal measurement at the HAWK.)

approximately 200 times higher since the shadowing entrance slit found in any classical spectrometer is not required. The short testing time which may become of essential importance in clinical and medical applications results from the working principle. The use of an interferometer allows the entire spectral range of interest to be observed at one point in time instead of a successive observation of single wavelengths and subsequent construction of the spectrum such as performed when working with classical spectrometer setups. Finally, the use of pilot lasers for distance measurement results in high accuracy of the wavenumber axis and the spectral resolution, respectively, of the resulting infrared spectrum. Here, an accuracy of 0.001 cm^{-1} can be obtained.

Fast measurement of infrared spectra as required in medical analysis of blood samples can furthermore be realised using the so-called attenuated total reflection (ATR) infrared spectroscopy. Here, the particular blood samples are brought in direct contact with an ATR-crystal, as shown in figure 4.7.

Total internal reflectance then occurs at the interface of the ATR-crystal and the blood sample. This allows the spectral detection and evaluation of the thinnest layers or very low sample volumes, respectively.

4.2 Microscopic measurement techniques

4.2.1 Confocal laser scanning microscopy

In the last decade, the use of confocal microscopy, most frequently also referred to as confocal laser scanning microscopy (CLSM), has been established for the

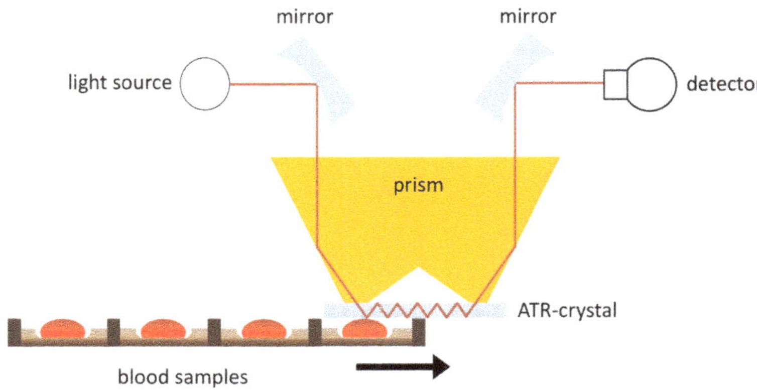

Figure 4.7. Principle of ATR infrared spectroscopy for the fast analysis of blood samples.

examination of tissue and could gradually replace classical microscopy in the future. For confocal laser scanning microscopy, the microscope image is composed of a number of sequential scans where each scan is realised on the basis of *in vitro* remission or fluorescence measurements. For this purpose, the raw beam of a laser source[9] is focussed where the focus diameter $2w_0$ amounts to

$$2w_0 \cong 2\lambda \frac{f}{D}. \tag{4.5}$$

Here, λ is the wavelength of the irradiation emitted by the laser source, f is the focal length of the optical system used, and D is its diameter[10]. The latter two parameters can also be expressed by the f-number, $f\#$, of the lens according to

$$f\# = \frac{f}{D}. \tag{4.6}$$

When working with aberration-corrected[11] microscope lenses with $f\# = 1$, a focus diameter of $2w_0 = 1$ μm can be obtained at a laser wavelength of $\lambda = 500$ nm. Such small focus diameters allow the spatial resolution and selective excitation of single cells or molecules. The resulting fluorescence signal is then collected and recorded by the confocal laser scanning microscope where the additional use of a photo multiplier, as shown in figure 4.8, allows time-resolved measurements.

For this purpose, a nitrogen laser-pumped dye laser can be used where the emission wavelength is adapted to the absorption maximum of the molecule of interest in order to induce efficient fluorescence. For instance, this approach has already been used for the time-resolved measurement of the energy transfer and the

[9] Usually, a dye laser source is employed for confocal laser scanning microscopy since such laser sources allow the realisation of a wide range of discrete laser wavelengths for inducing fluorescence.

[10] In optical science and engineering, the diameter of an optical system is also known as the aperture.

[11] Every optical system exhibits optical aberrations, i.e. spherical aberration, chromatic aberration, coma, astigmatism, Petzval field curvature and distortion. For imaging at high quality and resolution, these aberrations have to be minimised in the course of the design and manufacturing of the optical system.

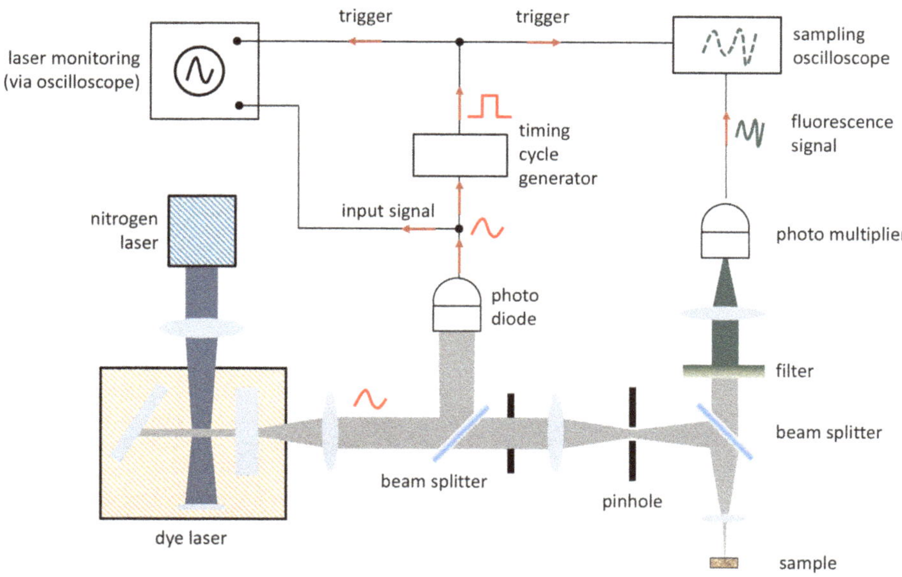

Figure 4.8. Schematic setup of a confocal laser scanning microscope for time-resolved measurements.

role of bases within deoxyribonucleic acid (DNA) molecules[12]. One of the main advantages of confocal laser scanning microscopy in comparison to classical microscopy is the possibility of measuring 3D images with a high depth resolution. This resolution is achieved by the working principle, as shown in figure 4.9: an image is acquired for a defined position of the pinholes with respect to the position of the laser focus. When shifting the focussed laser beam towards the sample, the arrangement is re-adjusted by high precision piezo controllers and the 3D model is successively generated on the basis of the particular slices measured for each step.

The thickness of a single measured slice is given by its full width at half maximum, FWHM, according to

$$\mathrm{FWHM} = \sqrt{\left(\frac{0.88 \cdot \lambda_{\mathrm{em}}}{[n - \sqrt{n^2 - \mathrm{NA}^2}]}\right)^2 + \left(\frac{\sqrt{2} \cdot n \cdot \mathrm{PH}}{\mathrm{NA}}\right)^2}. \tag{4.7}$$

Here, λ_{em} is the emission wavelength, PH is the diameter of the pinhole in the object space (see figure 4.9), n is the index of refraction of the surrounding medium (either air or an immersion liquid, compare figure 2.9 in section 2.2.2), and NA is the numerical aperture of the microscope lens. Such a distinct definition of the thickness of a measured slice is not possible when using classical light microscopes. This is due to the fact that here, sharp imaging exclusively occurs within the depth of focus of the microscope lens. This parameter is subject to wave-optical influences and phenomena, leading to a superposition of sharp optical signals from the actual focal point and blurred ones from neighbouring areas. A sample can thus not be

[12] Here, acridine was used as the tracer dye.

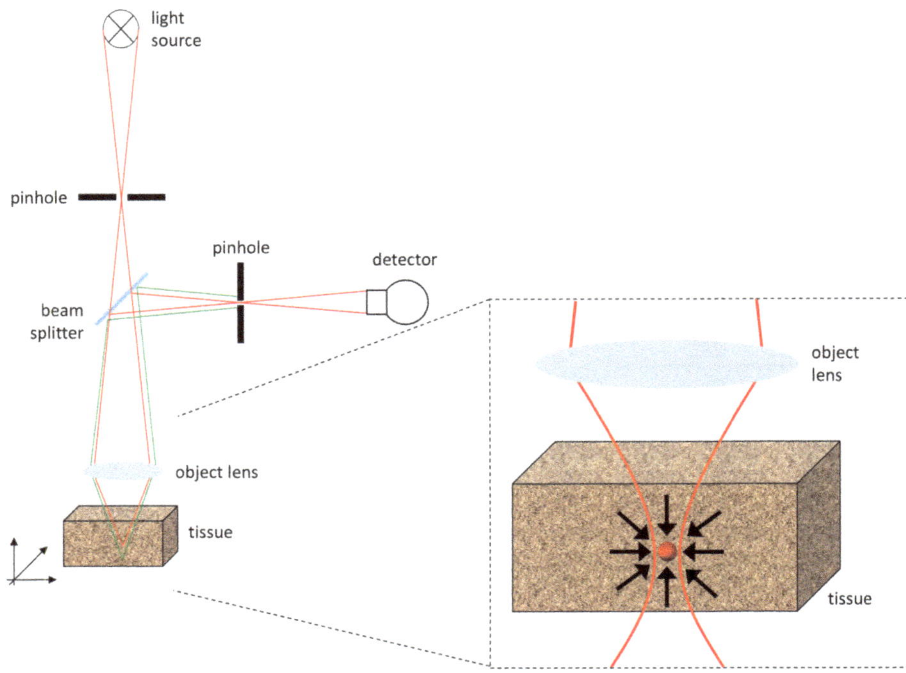

Figure 4.9. Basic setup of a confocal laser scanning microscope (LSM).

sliced optically into single and well-defined sections of interest. This fact shows the main advantage of a confocal laser scanning microscope in comparison to a classical microscope. Further advantageous features are the continuous and digital imaging, the comparatively high image contrast, the 3D image information and sectional images as well as the high sensitivity and efficiency.

4.2.2 Stimulated emission depletion microscopy

A stimulated emission depletion (STED) microscope is a special type of fluorescence microscope. In contrast to a classical optical microscope, its resolution is not limited by diffraction. As a result of the physical diffraction limit, the detection of very small structures with diameters d in the range of half the used wavelength λ[13] is impossible when working with optical microscopes. The minimum detectable diameter d is given by the Abbe equation according to

$$d = \frac{\lambda}{2 \cdot n \cdot \sin \alpha}. \quad (4.8)$$

Here, n is the index of refraction of the surrounding medium and α is the aperture angle of the used microscope lens. This inter-relationship is visualised and clarified in figure 4.10.

[13] For instance, the lateral resolution of a confocal microscope amounts to approximately 200 nm.

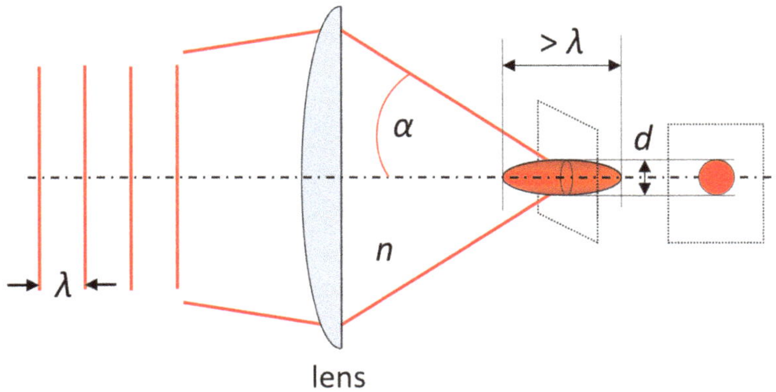

Figure 4.10. Visualisation of the Abbe equation.

The physical diffraction limit and the limit in detectable structure size, respectively, is avoided by the use of STED microscopes[14] which are based on the so-called RESOLFT[15] principle where the controlled switching off of selected fluorescence dyes allows the resolution to be increased significantly by reducing the fluorescing focal spot size as follows. Basically, a STED microscope is based on a florescence microscope setup. A focussed laser beam thus excites dye molecules within a biological sample. Once excitation of these dyes has occurred, the sample is irradiated by a second laser beam, also referred to as switch off beam, as shown in figure 4.11.

This second beam suppresses the excited molecules before a fluorescence signal is emitted. It features a specific beam profile where the laser intensity is not normally or Gaussian distributed. It can rather be described by a ring-shaped distribution[16].

This ring, as provided by the second laser, is placed around the spot of the first laser. As a consequence, only the fluorescence signal of a few molecules in the centre of the first laser which is not covered by the ring-shaped beam of the second laser is detected. As shown in figure 4.12, the microscope's resolution can then be increased (i.e. the detectable lateral structure size can be reduced) by increasing the intensity I of the second laser beam [4, 5].

In principle, a laser focus in the size range of a molecule can be obtained by STED microscopy where the saturation intensity I_{sat} of the used flourophore has to be taken into account according to

$$2w_0 = \frac{\lambda}{2 \cdot n \cdot \sin\alpha \cdot \sqrt{\dfrac{I}{I_{\text{sat}}}}}. \tag{4.9}$$

STED microscopy thus opens a wide field of novel possibilities for analyses in biophotonics and medical research.

[14] Applying STED microscopy, a lateral resolution of merely 2.4 nm was already reported in [3].

[15] RESOLFT is the abbreviation for REversible Saturable OpticaL Fluorescence Transitions.

[16] In laser physics, a ring-shaped laser beam is described by the specification TEM_{01*} which indicates the distribution of the transverse electromagnetic mode (TEM). This mode is also referred to as doughnut mode. A perfect rotational-symmetric and Gaussian distributed laser beam is specified by TEM_{00}.

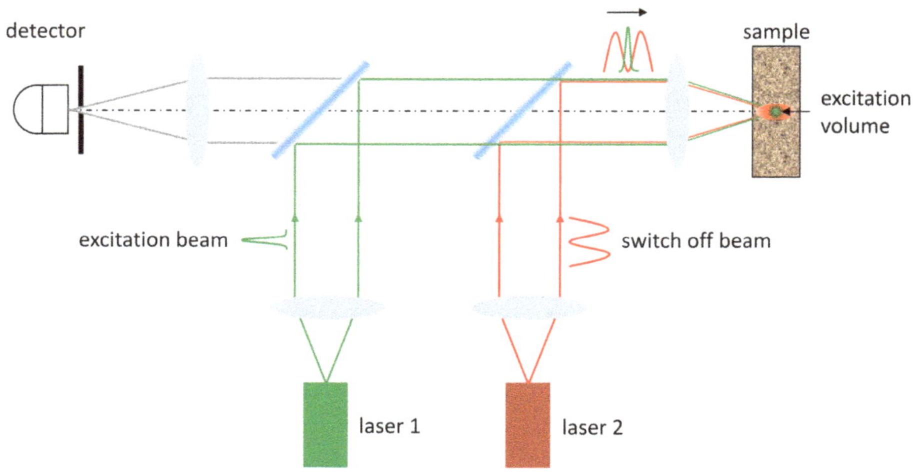

Figure 4.11. Basic setup of a STED microscope (adapted from [6]).

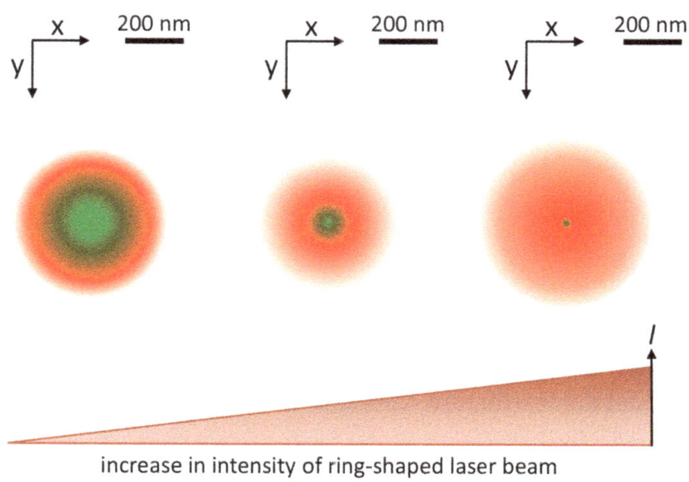

Figure 4.12. Principle of STED microscopy; fluorescence is induced by incident laser irradiation (green circle = exciting focus) and immediately suppressed by a second, ring-shaped laser beam (red circle = switch off beam). The size of the fluorescing focus decreases with increasing intensity *I* of the switch off beam.

4.3 Wave front sensing

Prior to the actual application of laser-assisted *in situ* keratomileusis (LASIK), as described in detail in section 5.3.2, an extensive and accurate characterisation of the eye concerned is mandatory. Since LASIK is basically the removal of material from the cornea, the shape and dimension of the material to be removed has to be characterised and specified in an initial step by measuring the present defective vision. This is made possible by the use of so-called Shack–Hartmann wave front sensors. Such sensors are robust and stable and merely consist of a micro lens array and a detector, usually a CCD[17] camera. The measurement principle of such a sensor can be described as follows: a bundle of collimated light rays can be described by a number of single light rays which propagate parallel to each other. The single light rays are thus orthogonal to a common plane. This plane is the wave front WF. In the case of laser irradiation with the wavelength λ and a constant phase function Φ, this wave front is given by

$$WF = \Phi \frac{\lambda}{2 \cdot \pi}. \tag{4.10}$$

The intensity and direction of propagation of a homogenous wave front and each involved single light ray is described by the so-called Poynting vector. This vector is given by the Cartesian product of the vector of the electric field and the magnetic field of a light wave[18]. From a mathematical or physical point of view, the area which is formed by perpendicular incidence of the Poynting vector of each single ray corresponds to the wave front. This approach even allows the description and specification of the wave front of incoherent light. The basic idea of a Shack–Hartmann sensor is to section a bundle of light rays with a certain diameter into a number of smaller bundles of light rays (as many and as small as possible). This can be realised by pinhole arrays or micro lens arrays. When using a micro lens array, the incoming bundle of light rays is sectioned into a number of sub-apertures[19] and additionally focussed. This effect increases the measurement accuracy as follows. For a plane wave front without any deformation, the focal point of each sub-aperture beam is imaged on a detector and gives an equidistant pattern of foci, as shown in figure 4.13(a). In contrast, a deformed wave front gives an irregular pattern of foci, see figure 4.13(b).

Taking the initial wave front as a reference, the resulting displacement between the foci can be determined in terms of its direction and amount (i.e. a vector). Considering the optical setup and its magnification, the wave front deformation can finally be constructed. It follows from the particularly measured displacements Δx of each sub-aperture beam which corresponds to an equivalent angle of inclination α between the optical axes of the measured beam and a reference beam produced by a wave front without any distortion, as shown in figure 4.14. For this purpose, the focal length f of the micro lenses which form the used micro lens array has to be taken into account according to

$$\Delta x = f \cdot \tan \alpha. \tag{4.11}$$

[17] CCD = charge-coupled device; within a CCD, an electrical charge is induced by incident light and subsequently converted into a signal.

[18] Remember that a light ray is merely a model which allows an easy and comprehensive characterisation of the direction of propagation of light. A more precise description of light is the model of a transversal electromagnetic wave. Here, the electric and the magnetic field are perpendicular to each other and the corresponding light ray is given by the base line of oscillation of both fields.

[19] In practice, an incoming bundle of light rays is sectioned into approximately 100–1000 sub-apertures, depending on the particular sensor setup and the required resolution.

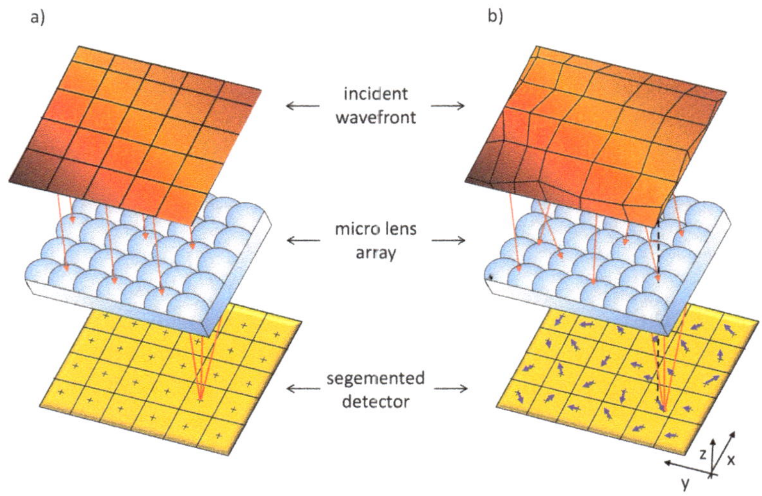

Figure 4.13. Functional principle of a Shack–Hartmann wave front sensor; an incident wave front is segmented into a number of sub-aperture beams by a micro lens array and each sub-aperture beam is focussed on a segmented detector. An undistorted or plane incident wave front provides an equidistant and regular pattern of foci on the detector (a), whereas a displacement of foci results in the case of a distorted wave front (b) (adapted from [7]).

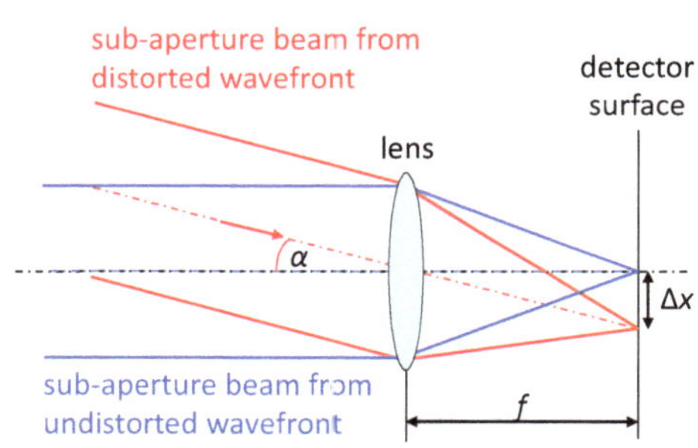

Figure 4.14. Visualisation of the displacement Δx of a focal point resulting for inclined incidence of light from the optical axis of a lens with the focal length f.

It should further be noted that the measured wave front must be continuously differentiable. Severe and local deformations of the wave front, for example steps which exceed the wavelength of light used for the measurement, as visualised in figure 4.15, cannot be calculated by the underlying mathematical models used for the evaluation of the measured wave front.

The measurement of defective vision and aberrations of the eye lens using Shack–Hartmann wave front sensors is shown in figure 4.16. The eye is irradiated with collimated laser light which is reflected at the retina. This means that the dioptric system of the eye[20] is crossed twice by the laser beam; it is thus a double-

[20] The dioptric system consists of all the involved optically-active and refracting components of the eye, i.e. the cornea, the anterior ocular chamber, the eye lens and the vitreous body.

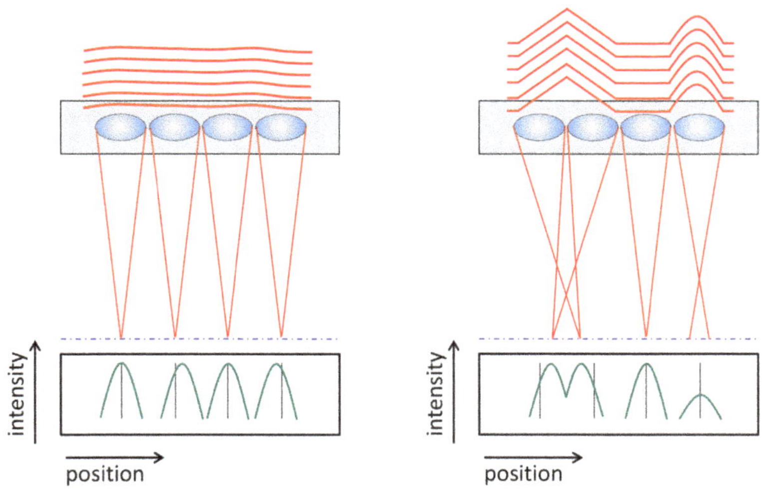

Figure 4.15. Conditions for the correct measurement of a wave front; slight wave front deformations can be evaluated (left), whereas severe and local deformations lead to the formation of non-interpretable signals on the detector (right).

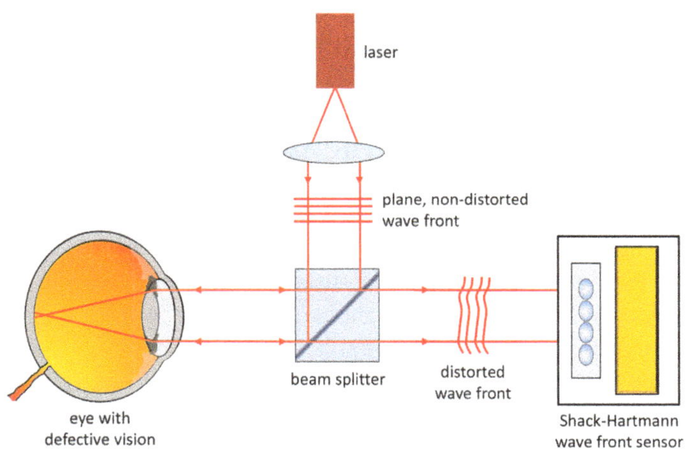

Figure 4.16. Shack–Hartmann wave front sensor-based setup for the determination of defective vision.

pass measurement principle with increased measurement accuracy. Based on the aberrations of the dioptric system detected in this way, a pattern for subsequent LASIK, i.e. a map of the current and the target surface shape of the cornea is generated.

The setup shown in figure 4.16 not only contains a Shack–Hartmann sensor, but also includes an interferometer[21] which is given by the light source (a laser with a

[21] The interferometer used here is a setup according to Fizeau, a special and robust type of common-path interferometer where the reference and measurement beam are not separated, but propagate along a common optical axis.

defined reference wave front), the beam splitter, and the retina which acts as mirror. The additional use of an interferometer becomes crucial since simple detectors such as CCD chips allow the measurement of intensity, but not the phase[22] of an incident light wave. This information is necessary for a distinct description of the defective vision.

4.4 Optical coherence tomography

Optical coherence tomography (OCT) is applied for the interior measurement and diagnosis of scattering samples, especially biological tissue layers with a high water content. Thanks to the use of light sources at low intensity in the range of some microwatts, OCT does not come along with critical radiation exposure in contrast to clinical radiology. It is thus a method of high relevance in medicine. In principle, OCT is quite comparable to diagnostic sonography where coherent broadband light from short pulse lasers, superluminescent diodes (SLED or SLD), or other suitable light sources is used instead of ultrasonic sound. This allows imaging with a high resolution of up to 0.5 μm[23], but a much smaller depth of measurement of approximately 2 mm in comparison to sonography due to scattering. Optical coherence tomography thus closes the gap between ultrasonic methods and confocal microscopy as shown in figure 4.17.

In the last decades, a number of different variations of optical coherence tomographic methods have been developed. The core element of most of these variations and the time-based standard OCT technique is a Michelson interferometer (compare the description of an FTIR spectrometer setup in section 4.1.2), as shown in figure 4.18.

The reference mirror in such an interferometer can be shifted. In this vein, any reference plane, i.e. a concentric circle where the circle centre is given by the point of beam splitting, see figure 4.18, can be realised. The signal detected by this setup is thus the scattered light coming from the sample layer which corresponds to the reference plane adjusted by the movable reference mirror. Consequently, an interferogram of this signal and the signal reflected by the reference mirror is formed by optical cross correlation of both arms. This allows the identification of the relative optical path lengths within the measured depth profile. When measuring the entire range of realisable reference planes, an A-scan[24] is obtained. The apposition of several A-scans during screening allows the generation of a two-dimensional image, the so-called B-scan[25]. Finally, a three-dimensional OCT scan is referred to as C-scan. In medical diagnosis, optical coherence tomography is mainly used in ophthalmology and dermatology, for example for the early detection of cancer. Here, the reflection at optical interfaces is detected in order to reconstruct a three-

[22] The phase of a light wave is the indirect information on its temporal and spatial state of oscillation at the moment of measurement.

[23] The resolution of optical coherence tomography is thus one to two orders of magnitude higher than for diagnostic sonography.

[24] Here, the abbreviation ‘A’ means ‘amplitude modulation’.

[25] In this context, ‘B’ means ‘brightness’.

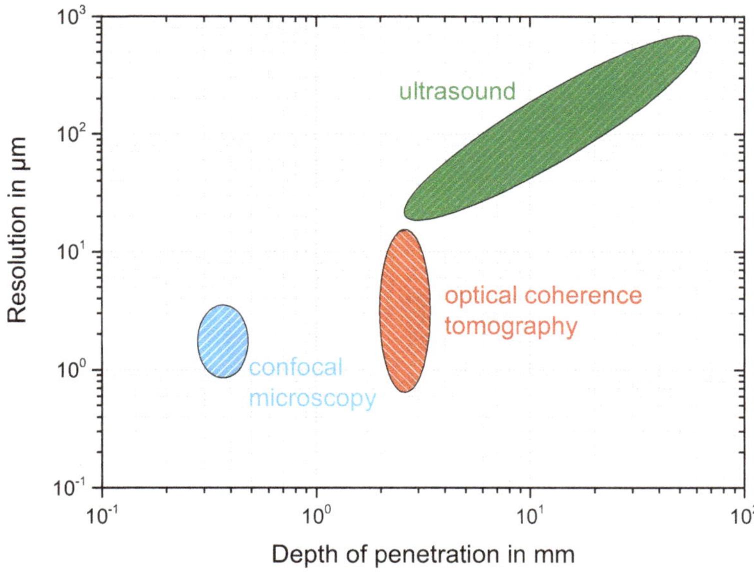

Figure 4.17. Comparison of the resolution and depth of measurement of confocal microscopy, optical coherence tomography (OCT) and ultrasonic methods. It turns out that the latter method features high depths of measurement, but comparatively poor resolution. The high coherence of the light sources used for OCT allows the realisation of high resolutions from 0.5 to 15 µm, but low depths of measurement of approximately 2–3 mm. The highest resolution in the sub-micrometre range and the lowest depth of measurement of some hundreds of micrometres is found for confocal microscopy.

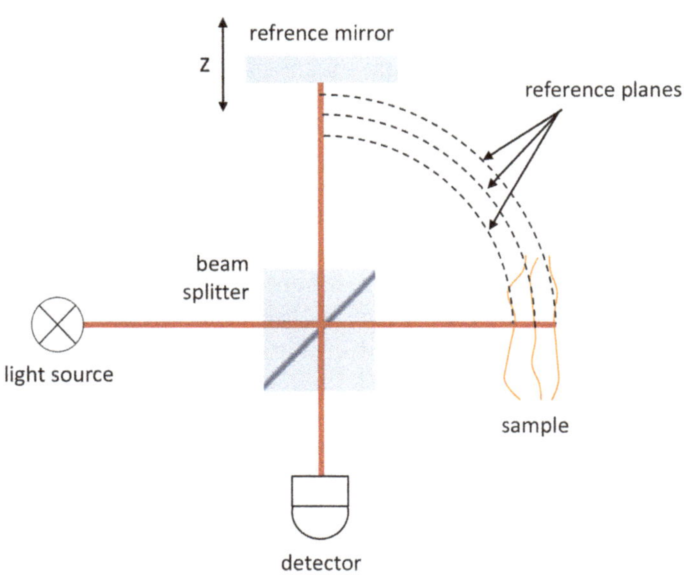

Figure 4.18. Setup of a Michelson interferometer consisting of a light source, a beam splitter device, a reference mirror and the sample.

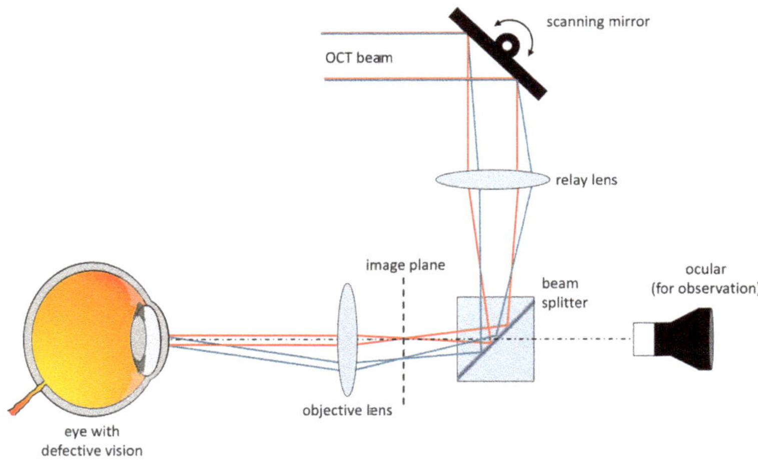

Figure 4.19. Schematic of an OCT setup for the three-dimensional examination of the ocular fundus.

dimensional C-scan. As an example, figure 4.19 shows an OCT setup for the examination of the ocular fundus.

In contrast to other techniques such as confocal microscopy, OCT allows the measurement of the fine layer structure of the retina, which exhibits a total thickness of only 250–300 μm, with high resolution[26]. Hence, the application of optical coherence tomography can be helpful for the detection of diseases of the retina which accompany an increase in thickness of the retina, the accumulation of fluid (i.e. the formation of oedema) or retinal detachment. This includes the formation of macular holes, diabetic retinopathy[27], glaucoma[28], and age-related macular degeneration (AMD). Such diseases cause severe sight disorders and even blindness in the most extreme and severe cases. It should finally be noted that OCT can easily be implemented into a number of existing diagnosis setups and thus even be applied intravascularly when introduced to endoscopes or catheters.

4.5 Pulse oximetry

The non-invasive method of pulse oximetry is used for monitoring the oxygen saturation within blood and tissue. It is thus a valuable diagnostic tool for the early recognition and therapy of low oxygen supply and oxygen deficiency. Decreased oxygen saturation causes hypoxia which may result in mental confusion or loss of consciousness and even reach potential life-threatening states[29] as indicated by a

[26] Regarding the examination of the human eye, optical non-contact measurements are of high hygienic and psychological relevance. First, the risk of infections is reduced significantly and second, mental stress of the patient is avoided to a large extent.

[27] Diabetes may cause circulatory disorder and accumulation of fluid within the retina.

[28] Glaucoma leads to creeping damage of the optic nerve which accompanies a reduction of the thickness of the retina. Optical coherence tomography could thus allow the diagnosis of this severe disease at an early stage.

[29] On average, mental dysfunctions occur at arterial oxygen saturation lower than 65%. Unconsciousness and more severe symptoms as well as low blood pressure can arise at arterial oxygen saturation levels lower than 55%.

cyanotic colour change of the patient due to desaturation. Against this background, pulse oximetry is an obligatory monitoring technique in intensive care and anaesthesia. In addition to oxygen saturation, this method allows the pulse frequency and eventual alternans of the heart to be detected. The setup of a pulse oximeter is quite simple[30]. It consists of a light source, usually diodes which emit red ($\lambda = 660$ nm) and infrared ($\lambda = 940$ nm) light, and a couple of photo detectors for the measurement of the intensity of light. These elements are arranged oppositely in a finger clip. This clip is fixed to an easily accessible body part such as for example a finger, a toe, or an earlobe. Pulse oximetry is based on two different measurement principles, spectrophotometry and photo-plethysmography. In the first case, the difference in absorption of oxygenated and deoxygenated haemoglobin is employed. The light emitted by the diodes (red and infrared) is measured by the detectors after passing the particular body part where the oximeter is fixed, as shown in figure 4.20. The resulting absorbance for each wavelength is then calculated and finally, the ratio of the absorbance of red light and infrared light is determined. This ratio corresponds to a certain value of oxygen saturation[31] and is thus the actual parameter of interest. This approach, spectrophotometry, could be referred to as an integrating method since the absorption is determined for all blood vessels by shining a light through them.

The method of dynamic photo-plethysmography allows selective measurement of the absorbance of the arterial blood. Here, the measured signal, obtained at an infrared illumination wavelength, for example 940 nm, is segmented in a continuous and a pulsed[32] one. The continuous fraction is related to venous and capillary blood, bones, abdomen, and tissue. As shown in figure 4.21, the pulsed absorption signal

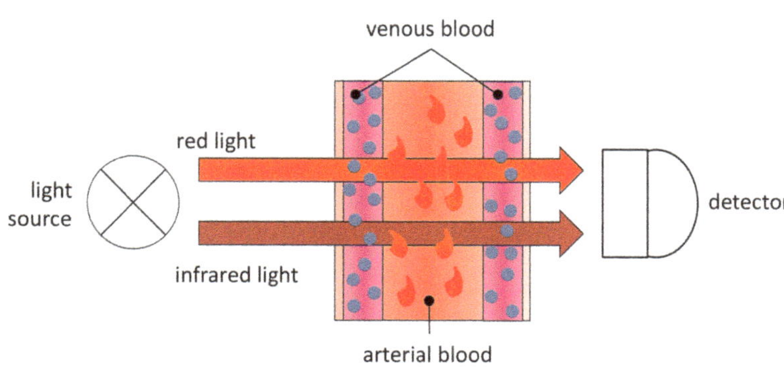

Figure 4.20. Measuring principle of a pulse oximeter.

[30] Due to the simple setup, a pulse oximeter is an extremely cost efficient medical measurement device; the sales price of a simple pulse oximeter for consumer markets is approximately 10–20 Euros.
[31] The required reference data are determined empirically in the course of studies with healthy probands and summarised in nomograms.
[32] This is made possible by the pulsing character of the cardiac cycle which results from its two parts when the heart is filled and emptied, respectively, The first part, filling, is referred to as diastole, the second, emptying, is called systole and is due to the heart's contraction.

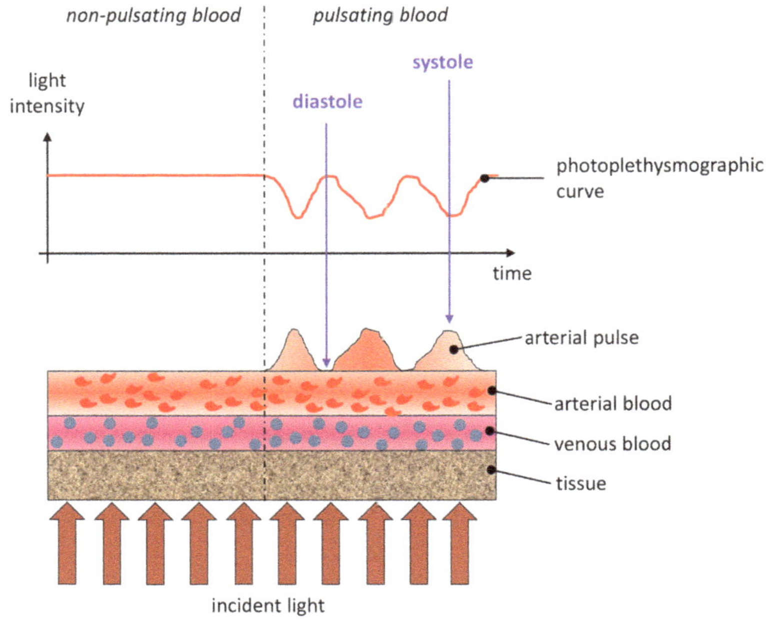

Figure 4.21. Principle of dynamic photo-plethysmography for the measurement of the absorbance of arterial blood on the basis of the two parts of the cardiac cycle, diastole and systole.

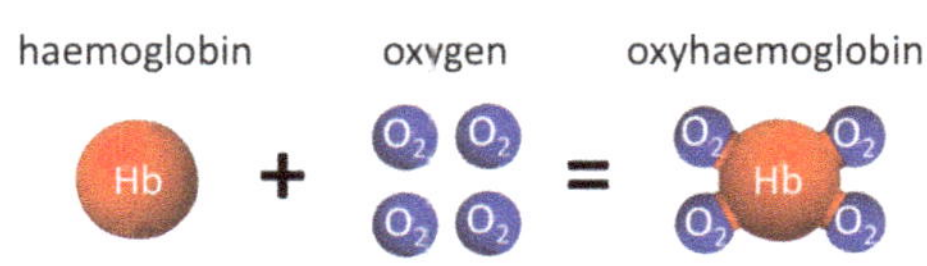

Figure 4.22. Visualisation of the uptake of oxygen molecules (O_2) by a haemoglobin molecule (Hb), resulting in the formation of fully saturated oxyhaemoglobin.

can finally be attributed to arterial blood. The measurement of the oxygen saturation of arterial blood provides information on the mean load of haemoglobin with oxygen. The maximum oxygen uptake of one haemoglobin molecule (Hb) is four oxygen molecules (O_2). This corresponds to a saturation of 100%, shown in figure 4.22. This bond is referred to as oxyhaemoglobin and is mainly found within arterial blood where about 1.5% of physically solved oxygen is existent additionally. Pulse oximetric measurements provide the mean saturation of haemoglobin molecules in arterial blood. However, it gives the peripheral oxygen saturation (S_pO_2), but not the actual venous oxygen saturation (S_vO_2) or the arterial oxygen saturation (S_aO_2),[33] which is indicated by the index 'p'[34].

[33] The standard value of the arterial oxygen saturation amounts to 96–100%.

[34] The index 'p' officially denotes 'peripheral' but is also sometimes used as the abbreviation for 'pulse oximetric'.

This index clearly demarcates an oxygen saturation value as determined via pulse oximetry from oxygen saturation measured at classical blood samples. The peripheral oxygen saturation is given by

$$S_pO_2 = \frac{HbO_2}{HbO_2 + Hb} \tag{4.12}$$

where HbO_2 is the concentration of oxygenated haemoglobin and Hb is the concentration of deoxygenated haemoglobin which exhibits free places for potential oxygen uptake and transport.

4.6 Synthetic aperture linking

Rheumatism is one of the most widespread diseases[35]. It covers a number of quite different musculoskeletal disorders, where pain and dysfunctions mainly occur at joints, sinews, muscles, and nerves. The main groups of rheumatic diseases including the particular sub-groups are listed is table 4.2.

For instance, the diagnosis of rheumatoid arthritis (RA) in its early state is not possible by conventional imaging methods [9, 10]. However, early detection is a mandatory condition for successful therapy. It is of notable relevance since RA is the most common inflammatory arthropathy of the connective tissue and occurs at finger joints in most cases. Even though the RA is not yet fully understood, its aetiopathology can be classified in four main states:

Table 4.2. Main groups of rheumatic diseases including the particular frequency and sub-groups [8].

Main group	Frequency	Sub-groups
Inflammatory rheumatic diseases	≈20%	Rheumatoid arthritis (RA) Rheumatic fever Ankylosing spondylitis (AS) Pararheumatic diseases, e.g. systemic lupus erythematosus (SLE), also known as lupus
Degenerative rheumatic diseases	≈40%	Osteoarthritis (OA) Degenerative alterations of the spinal column (spinal osteochondrosis) and other cartilages
Extra-articular rheumatic diseases	≈40%	Muscle rheumatism Bursitis Tendinitis and tendovaginitis Panniculitis

[35] For instance, 1.5 million of the 80 million residents in Germany suffer from rheumatism.

- Release of antigens due to an autoimmune reaction to bacteria, virus etc
- Aggressive adenoid vegetation of the synovial membrane and alteration of the synovia
- Destruction of the cartilage layer between the bones by lysosomal enzymes
- Adhesion of bones after complete destruction of cartilage.

The early stage of this process cannot be detected by the evaluation of radiographs since here, the contrast follows from the tissue density. As a consequence, inflammatory rheumatic alterations can only be detected at a later stage, i.e. after the destruction of cartilage and the accompanying alteration of the tissue density. For the identification of early-stage phenomena such as an alteration of the synovia and an early diagnosis of RA, other techniques such as the so-called synthetic aperture linking (SAL) have to be applied [11, 12]. This method can be performed on the basis of two different approaches: time-resolved measurement and intensity modulated measurement.

Time-resolved synthetic aperture linking

In the case of time-resolved synthetic aperture linking, the goal is to gain information on an irradiated tissue volume from changes in absorption which correspond to the morphology and geometry of the tissue and the content of different substances such as oxygen or reduced nicotinamide adenine dinucleotide (NADH). However, the determination of absorption is based on the measurement of transmission which becomes complicated in the case of scattering media. As shown in figure 4.23, the photons detected in the course of transmission measurements might have covered notably different distances, i.e. optical paths due to scattering and may not even have interacted with the absorber of interest.

As a result of such scattering, the particular photon paths feature different optical distances and travel times, respectively, giving rise to a time delay between the detected single photons. This effect is applied in order to separate photons which were subject to either high or moderate scattering where the latter contain the best spatial information. In practice, a tissue sample is irradiated by a short laser pulse with a pulse duration of some picoseconds. When crossing the tissue

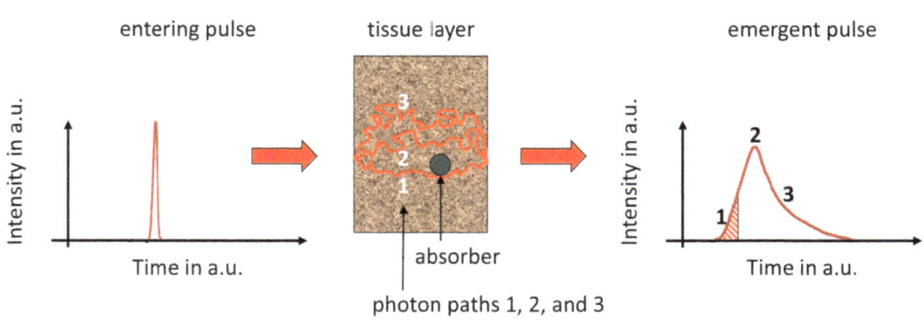

Figure 4.23. Visualisation of the underlying mechanism for time-resolved synthetic aperture linking; an entering laser pulse is scattered within a tissue layer, resulting in the formation of different photon paths and a temporal stretching of the laser pulse (adapted from [13]).

material, this pulse is temporally stretched, as shown in figure 4.23(right), its pulse duration is then in the range of one to two nanoseconds. This delay distribution strongly depends on the absorption coefficient, the scattering coefficient, the anisotropy factor (see section 3.1.1) and the thickness of the tissue. The stretched pulse can finally be interpreted as follows. The rising edge of the pulse represents photons which were not or insignificantly scattered (photon path and pulse position 1 in figure 4.23). The pulse centre and its neighbouring zone contains information on snaking or curling photons which were scattered along a zigzag-shaped path around the principal direction of propagation (photon path and pulse position 2 in figure 4.23). Finally, photons which were subject to strong scattering are found in the falling edge of the stretched pulse (photon path and pulse position 3 in figure 4.23). The evaluation of such a stretched pulse is carried out by defining a certain optimum temporal window of detection, the so-called gate width. Since the photons of interest are found in the rising edge, this window usually includes this part of the pulse. However, the measurement of thicker tissue samples with a thickness of some centimetres requires extensive technical equipment since in this case, non-scattered photons cannot be detected and the share of snaking photons merely accounts for 1% of the entire pulse signal. Nowadays, time-resolved synthetic aperture linking can thus be performed under laboratory conditions, but is not applicable for routine clinical examination. Here, the approach of intensity modulated measurements gains in importance.

Intensity modulated synthetic aperture linking

Intensity modulated synthetic aperture linking is based on the evaluation of the amplitude and phase shift of continuously irradiated and amplitude modulated light [14]. Here, amplitude modulation is performed in order to realise a wavelike expansion of the exciting light within the scattering sample, i.e. tissue. The resulting photon-density-wave can basically be described by a wave with a certain phase velocity and wavelength. Both parameters depend on the modulation frequency and the optical properties of the tissue and thus alter when crossing tissue of a different composition. As shown in figure 4.24, the amplitude and the phase shift of the detected light change when an absorber within a scattering medium is irradiated with amplitude modulated light. The detected signal thus contains information on the position of the absorber.

An increased phase shift and loss in intensity or amplitude is found if an absorber is placed in the middle of the light path of the scattered light. In contrast, a reduced phase shift, corresponding to a decreased mean travel path of the photons, is observed if the scattered light grazes an absorber. The detected signal consequently contains information on physical phenomena such as diffraction, reflection and refraction which results in a change in the attenuation and travel time of photons. With respect to time-resolved synthetic aperture linking, the main advantage of this approach is the possibility of continuous and easy measurement with standard equipment. Here, no short pulse lasers and the appropriate detection units are

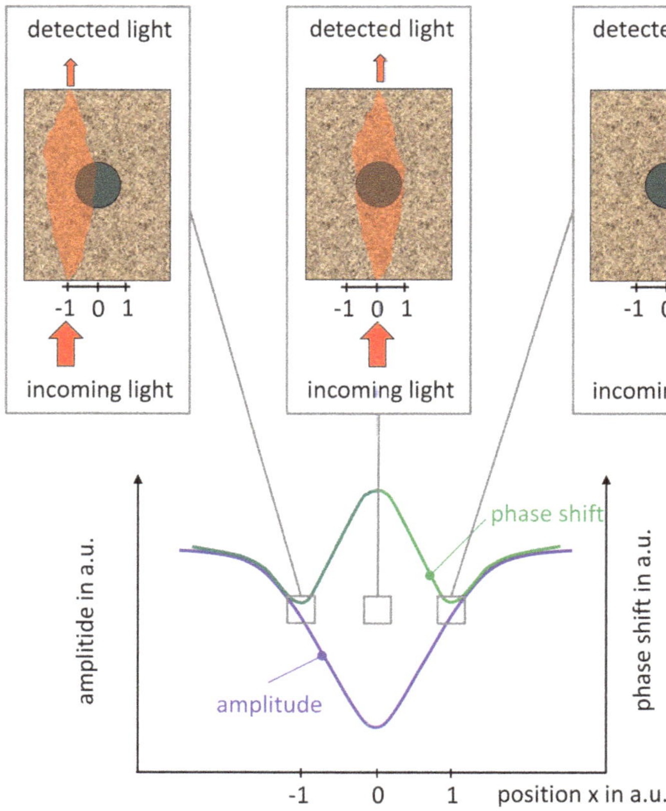

Figure 4.24. Visualisation of the underlying mechanism for intensity modulated synthetic aperture linking; a scattering medium is irradiated with amplitude modulated light which is scattered and additionally attenuated by an absorber (green circle). The evaluation of the resulting change in amplitude and the phase shift allows the optical properties of the examined medium to be determined (adapted from [13]).

required. The basic setup of such a continuous wave illumination system used for the early diagnosis of rheumatoid arthritis (RA) is shown in figure 4.25.

Figure 4.26 shows an example of scattering characteristics of an articular capsule and synovia in the healthy and early diseased state as measured by intensity modulated synthetic aperture linking. Here, a general increase in the effective scattering coefficient can be identified for the measured wavelengths in the red and near infrared spectral range.

To a certain extent, this also applies for the absorption coefficient, as shown in figure 4.27. Obvious changes are especially found around an observation wavelength of approximately 675 nm where an increase in tissue absorption can be identified. In contrast, the pathological impact on scattering and absorption at a wavelength of 905 nm can be neglected. It can thus be summarised that this approach is suitable for the early diagnosis of rheumatoid arthritis by the detection of changes of the optical properties of affected capsules and synovia.

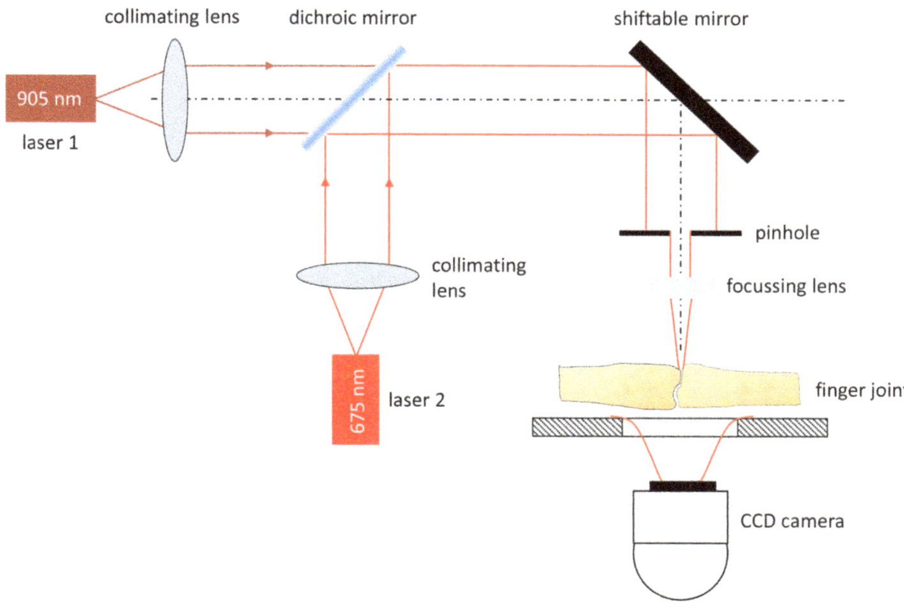

Figure 4.25. Continuous wave illumination system for the early diagnosis of RA based on two lasers for illumination at the two wavelengths of interest 675 nm and 906 nm (adapted from [11]).

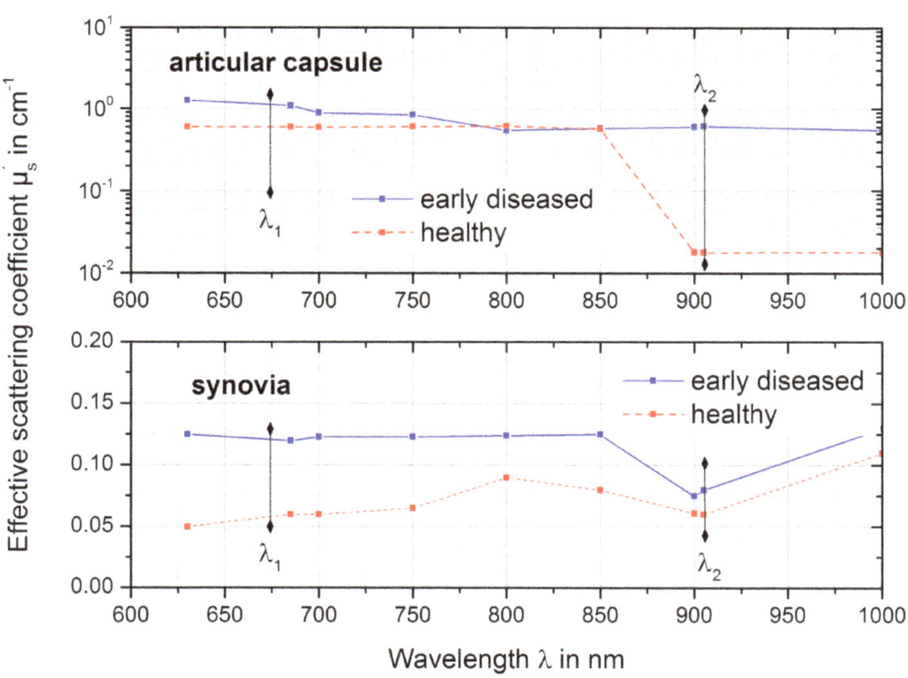

Figure 4.26. Effective scattering coefficient $\acute{\mu}_s$ of articular capsule (top) and synovia (bottom) in the healthy and early diseased state (adapted from [13]).

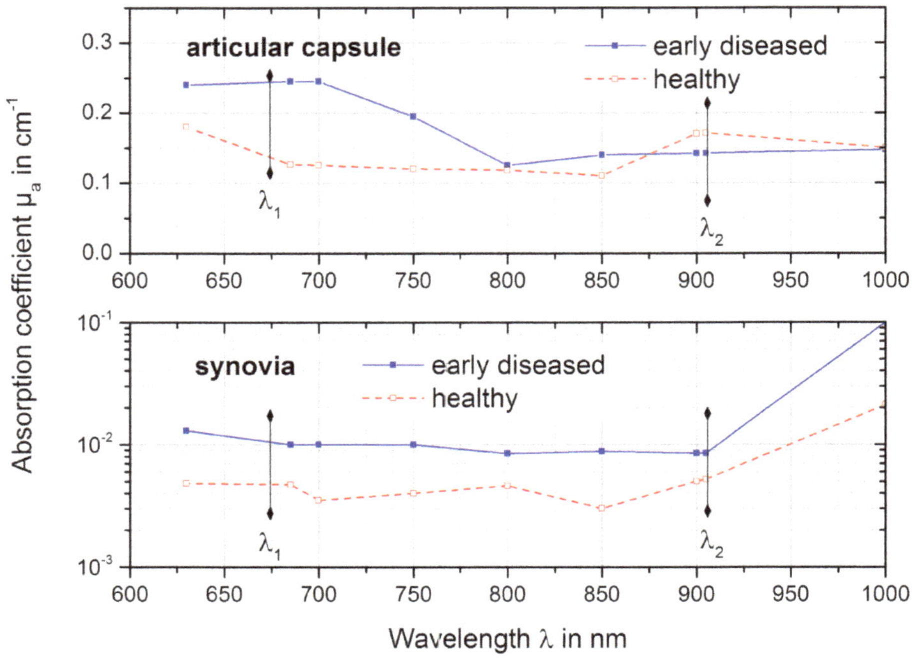

Figure 4.27. Absorption coefficient μ_a of articular capsule (top) and synovia (bottom) in the healthy and early diseased state (adapted from [13]).

4.7 Optical capnography

In general, capnography is the measurement and graphical displaying of the time-dependence of the partial pressure and concentration of carbon dioxide within a patient's exhalation air. Currently, two measurement methods, infrared spectroscopy and mass spectroscopy[36], are employed for this purpose in clinical applications where infrared spectroscopy represents the commonly used one. It is mainly applied for monitoring surgical interventions. Here, the exhalation air of a patient under anaesthetic is evaluated by an optical setup[37]. The composition of inhalation air and exhalation air is listed in table 4.3. The comparison in table 4.3 shows that approximately 5% of the inhaled oxygen is consumed and that carbon dioxide is generated within the human body, as shown by the increase of the carbon dioxide content in exhalation air by the same value. The molecular composition of the exhaled air is a suitable indicator for the optimum dose rate of narcotics during surgical intervention under general anaesthesia. Since this composition is given by the ratio of the concentrations of nitrogen, oxygen, and carbon dioxide, it can easily be measured

[36] Mass spectroscopy is not an optical measurement method. It is rather based on the detection of the masses of particles within a sample volume where the particular particle, i.e. molecule or cluster, is identified by its mass and the composition of the sample volume is derived from the measured mass distribution function.

[37] Here, two different main approaches for infrared spectroscopic measurement are used, the side stream method and the main stream method.

via optical capnography in real time. In order to increase its detection sensitivity, a so-called multiple pass setup, as shown in figure 4.28, can be used.

Here, the measuring laser beam is reflected between two mirrors and passes the sample gas, which is placed between those mirrors, several times. The actual detection and measurement is based on the principle of Raman spectroscopy[38]. The detectors which are arranged perpendicular to the reflected laser beams are thus

Table 4.3. Typical composition of inhalation air (i.e. normal atmosphere) and exhalation air.

Compound	Content in inhalation air in %	Content in exhalation air in %	Difference in %
Nitrogen (N_2)	78	78	0
Oxygen (O_2)	20.96	16	−4.96
Carbon dioxide (CO_2)	0.04	5	+4.96
Inert gases, e.g. argon (Ar)	1	1	0

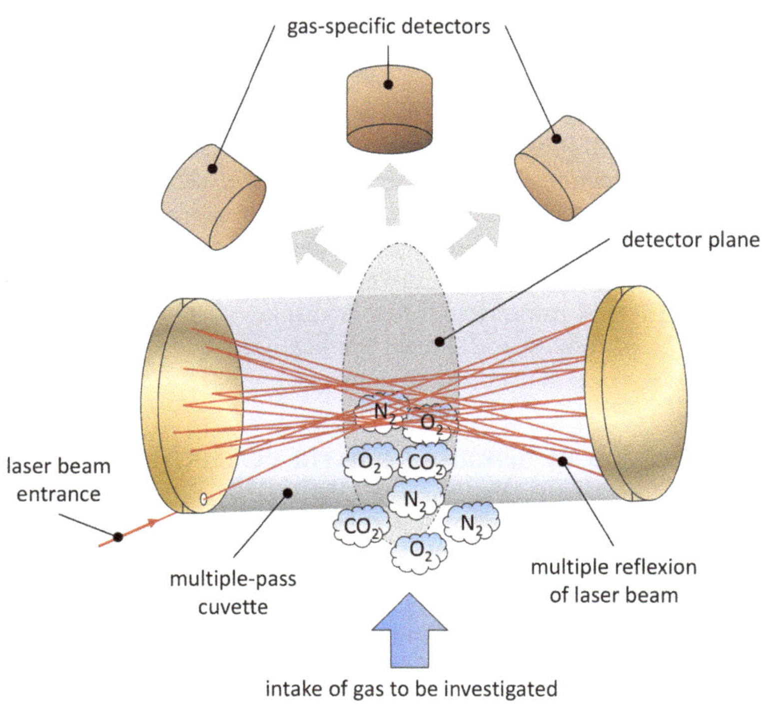

Figure 4.28. Multiple pass cell for increasing the sensitivity of an optical capnography setup.

[38] Raman spectroscopy is the spectroscopic investigation of any medium on the basis of inelastic scattering (Raman scattering) of light and allows detecting vibrational, rotational, and other low-frequency modes of molecules.

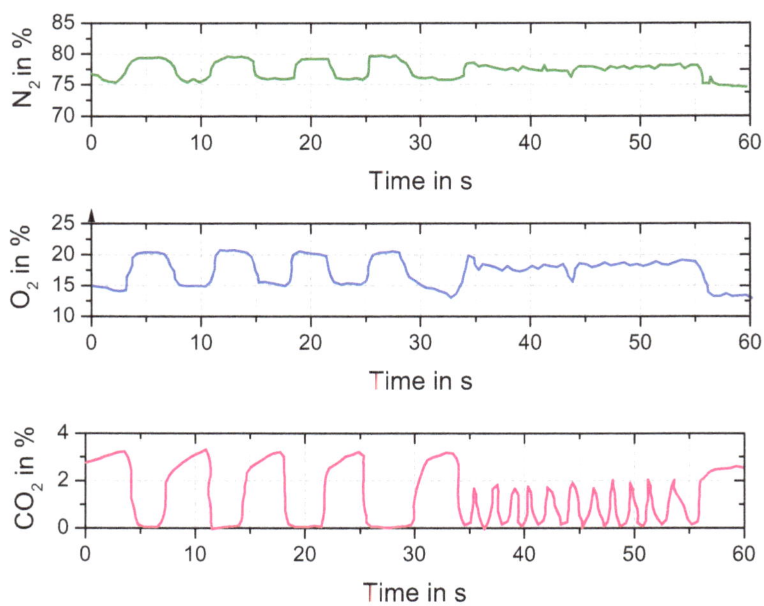

Figure 4.29. Concentration of nitrogen (N_2, top), oxygen (O_2, middle), and carbon dioxide (CO_2, bottom) of the exhaled air at different respiratory rates.

equipped with special filters. These filters feature high transmission for single Raman lines of molecules and thus allow increases in the measurement accuracy and reduction in the detection limit by improving the signal-to-noise ratio. The composition of the gas which is analysed by such a setup then follows from the ratio of the intensities of the measured Raman lines. The sensitivity of this method is shown in figure 4.29. Here, the temporal variation of the composition of exhaled air of a patient at different respiratory rates is displayed. Due to its accuracy, this method is not only of interest for clinical applications, but also for other purposes such as field sobriety tests during traffic controls.

4.8 Photoactivation of hematoporphyrin derivative

Photoactivation of hematoporphyrin derivative (HpD) is a comparatively novel method for the diagnosis and treatment of tumours which even allows devitalising tumour cells. It is thus a photodynamic therapy method, based on the activation of the fluorescent HpD. This substance is watered down and injected intravenously. The disintegration time of HpD amounts to 2–4 days in normal cells and may be stored for a longer period in cancer cells. When irradiated with ultraviolet laser irradiation, such tissue emits a characteristic fluorescence signal which allows the detection of cancer cells, as shown by the example in figure 4.30. In practice, fluorescence is mainly induced by nitrogen (N_2) lasers with an emission wavelength of approximately 337 nm. In order to isolate the HpD fluorescence from other fluorescence signals of normal cells that may arise, several filters are placed in the beam path [15, 16].

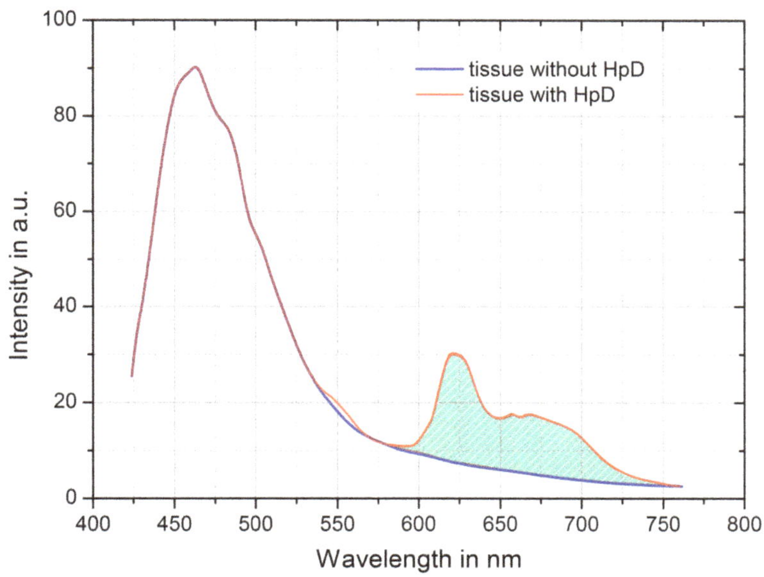

Figure 4.30. Fluorescence spectrum of pure tissue (blue line) and tissue two days after the injection of HpD (red line), visualising the additional HpD fluorescence signal (hatched area (adapted from [17]).

Another effect occurs if HpD is irradiated by red light at a wavelength of 620–640 nm. In this case, HpD is excited and reacts with the surrounding oxygen molecules. Normally, oxygen is existent in its ground state, i.e. the oxygen triplet, but is excited to the singlet oxygen. This high energy form of oxygen is toxic for tissue and thus attacks the surrounding cells, as shown in figures 4.31 and 4.32. This method consequently allows a selective disintegration of tumour cells and has already been applied successfully for the devitalisation of oesophageal cancer and skin carcinoma as well as other tumours which are otherwise difficult to access without any invasive surgery.

4.9 Flow cytometry

Flow cytometry[39] is a comparatively novel technique which is applied for the differentiation of particles or cells on the basis of fluorescence. For this purpose, particles or cells are solved in a carrier liquid and prepared by suitable fluorescent tracer dyes, i.e. fluorophores or fluorochromes, as shown in figure 4.33.

The liquid sample material then passes slowly[40] through a sample chamber made of glass, the flow cell, and fluorescence is induced by incident focussed laser irradiation. Due to the small diameter of the inner channel of the used flow cells and the accompanying formation of a sheath and hydrodynamic focussing of the

[39] Flow cytometry is sometimes also referred to as fluorescent activated cell sorting (FACS). This term is a registered trademark (registered by Becton–Dickinson).

[40] The flow rate typically ranges from 10 to 60 μl $\min^{-1}$.

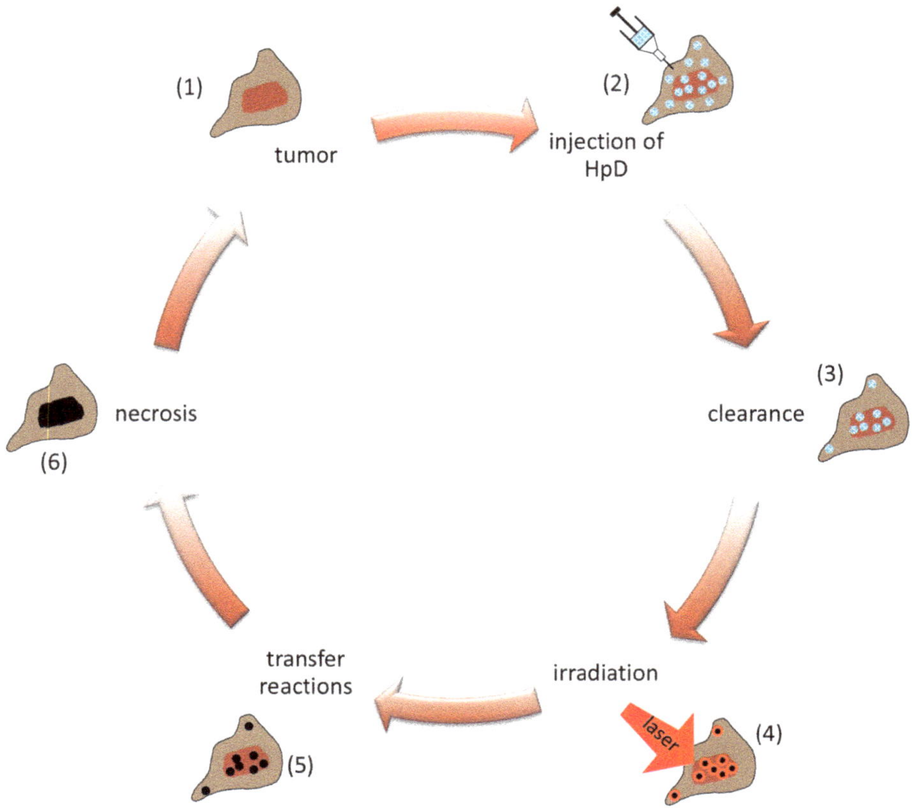

Figure 4.31. Example for a photodynamic therapy on the basis of photoactivation of hematoporphyrin derivative (HpD) and its photochemical impact on tissue (adapted from [17]).

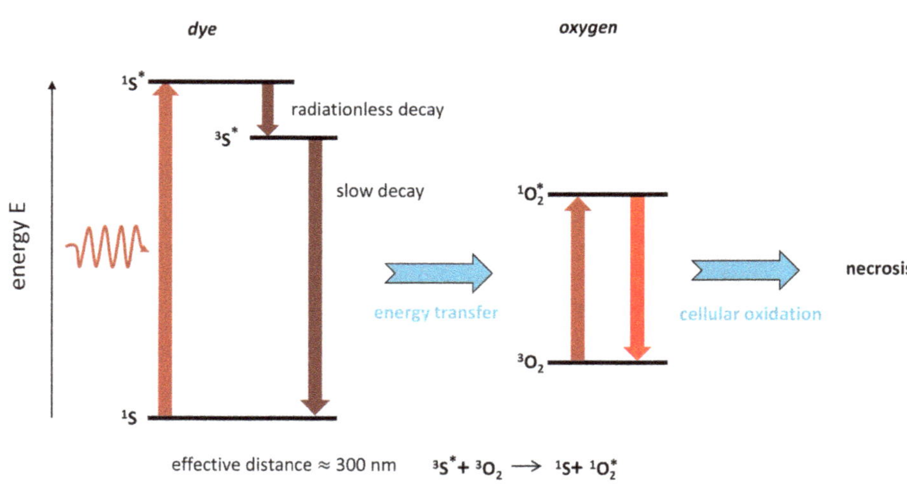

Figure 4.32. Process of the photodynamic therapy shown in figure 4.31 on the basis of the term diagrams of the involved species (adapted from [18]).

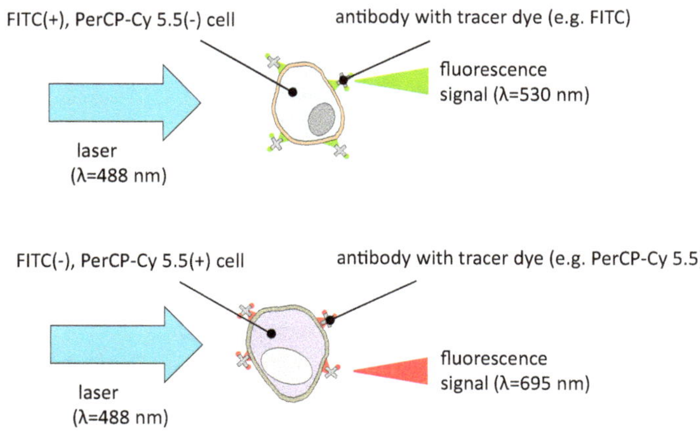

Figure 4.33. Principle of preparation of cells with fluorescent tracer dyes and formation of fluorescence signals due to incident laser light.

liquid sample medium, single particles and cells can be detected, as shown in figure 4.34.

This allows the quantitative analysis of the physical and molecular properties of intact cells at the highest flexibility. For this purpose, the scattering of incident laser light and fluorescence of tracer dyes are detected at the same time, as shown in figure 4.35.

Here, the liquid sample flow passes a focused laser beam, resulting in scattering and the formation of fluorescence signals. The fluorescence forward scatter (FSC) signal allows the determination of the size of the measured particle or cell[41]. The fluorescence side scatter (SSC) signal which is perpendicular to the FSC contains information on the cell granularity, the structure of its core and the wavelength-dependent fluorescence which corresponds to a clearly defined type of particle or cell. For instance, this allows the number of bound antibodies or a cell's DNA concentration to be detected. The fluorescence forward and side scatter are moreover suitable for the differentiation of blood cells. The sensitivity of this method mainly depends on the preparation of the cells and the optical system of the imaging setup. In some cases, special solutions for preparing the liquid sample which are adapted to, and optimised for, the particular imaging system of different conventional flow cytometers are available. In order to evaluate the wavelength-dependent information of the SSC signal, dichroic mirrors[42] and pass filters (see figure 4.33) which are adapted to the used tracer dyes are employed, as shown in figure 4.36.

[41] This is made possible since the angular distribution of scattered light is directly linked to the size or volume of the scattering objects. Depending on the used flow cytometer, the minimum measurable cell size ranges from 500 nm to 1 μm. However, scattering is not only attributed to the cell size, but also to the surface structure and roughness of a cell where a higher surface roughness results in higher scattering.

[42] A dichroic mirror features high transmittance for a first and high reflectance for a second wavelength of interest. It thus allows one to separate (or combine) those wavelengths in terms of direction of propagation.

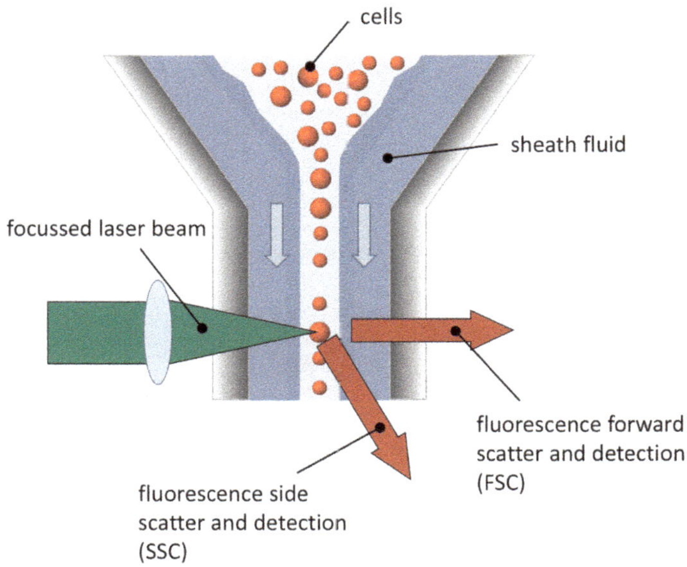

Figure 4.34. Principle of flow cytometry; particles and cells are brought in suspension and pass a focussed laser beam which induces fluorescence, the actually measured signal of interest, which can be categorised into fluorescence forward scatter (FSC) and fluorescence side scatter (SSC).

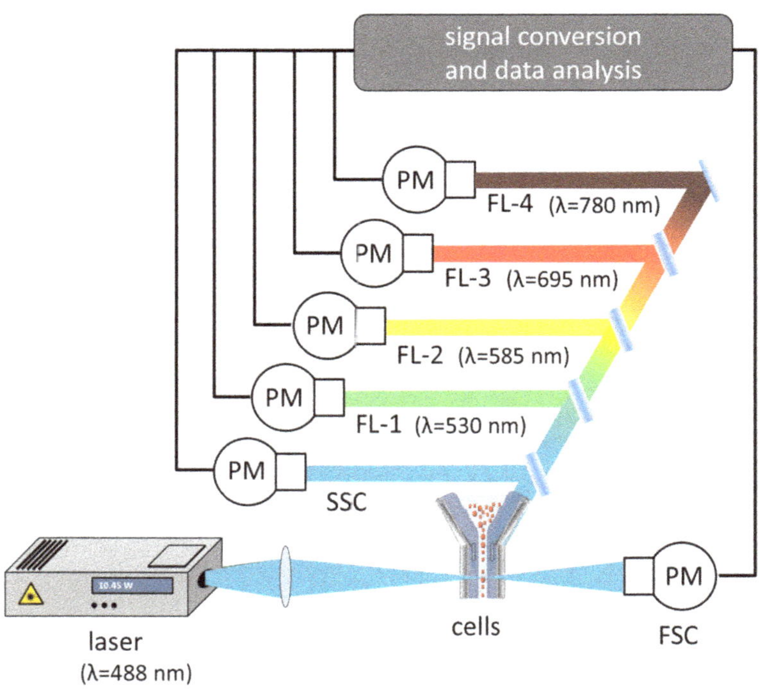

Figure 4.35. Basic setup of a flow cytometer for the detection of FSC and SSC via photomultipliers (PM) and for the spectral segmentation of the SSC signal into single fluorescence signals (FL) (adapted from [19]).

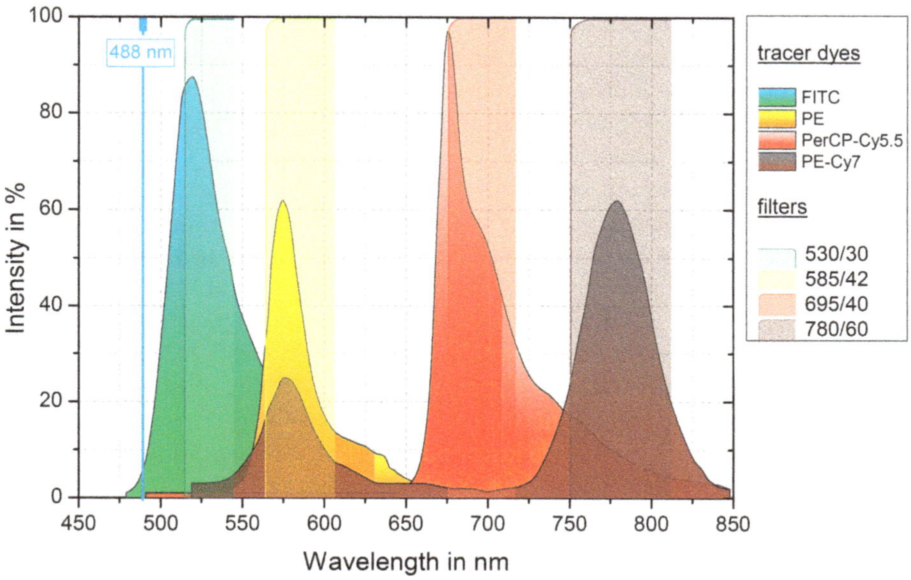

Figure 4.36. Overview of the fluorescence spectrum (curves) and filters (rectangles) of commercial fluorescent tracer dyes. (Data taken from BD Fluorescence Spectrum Viewer.)

Table 4.4. Standardised consecutive numbering of photo detectors of a flow cytometer including the corresponding wavelengths of the fluorescence signals resulting for an excitation wavelength of 488 nm (compare figure 4.35).

Number	Wavelength of fluorescence signal in nm
FL-1	530
FL-2	585
FL-3	695
FL-4	780

The detected quasi-monochromatic signals are then detected via photomultipliers which convert the incident light into electric signals which are evaluated and give the final result of the measurement. According to a standardised nomenclature, the used photo detectors are consecutively numbered, as listed in table 4.4 and shown in figure 4.36.

4.10 Laser-induced fluorescence for early recognition of caries

In addition to periodontitis, caries is the most widespread infectious disease. In the last few decades, the prevalence of caries is notably on the decline thanks to prophylactic actions and techniques such as fluoridation of dentifrices. However, it is still a problem and according to a survey presented by the American Dental Association (ADA) in 2001, approximately 90% of the US-American population suffered from treated or untreated caries. Even in the case of routine preventive dental examinations caries may be missed due to the fact that it occurs at interdental spaces or at the rim of chewing surfaces[43] which are difficult to access optically. Further, caries is often hidden under the adamantine that may macroscopically exhibit an (apparently) intact surface.

Here, laser-based fluorescence methods have turned out to be powerful tools which provide supplementary information and complete visual examination or radiographs. As listed in table 4.5, the additional use of such techniques allows the detection of caries more frequently, even at its early stage. At this stage, the affected adamantine or dentine is demineralised. In the course of progressive caries, the adamantine is then discoloured and finally collapses. At this later stage, caries can indeed be detected visually, but an extensive restoration of the affected tooth or even root canal therapy may become necessary.

For early recognition of caries via laser-induced fluorescence, a tooth is illuminated with laser light at a wavelength of 655 nm, as shown in figure 4.37. At the same time, the resulting fluorescence signal is detected and evaluated[44]. With respect to intact and unaffected adamantine and dentine, an eventual demineralisation and carious alternation would then be discovered on the basis of the fluorescence signal, see figure 4.38. This signal is proportional to the demineralisation of the tooth material; its wavelength amounts to 680 nm at the above-mentioned excitation wavelength. The emitted fluorescent light thus exhibits a slightly longer wavelength of the incident light which initiates the mechanisms of fluorescence.

The main advantage of this technique is given by the use of collimated laser beams with extremely small diameters. Laser irradiation can thus enter very small fissures which may not be accessed with any mechanical probe, as shown in figure 4.39. The possible depth of measurement amounts to 1.5–2 mm, depending on the diameter of the particular fissure.

Table 4.5. Success rates of different techniques for the detection of caries [20, 21].

Technique	Success rate
Visual inspection	≈49%
Radiographs (bitewing)	≈55%
Electric caries monitoring[45]	≈85%
Laser fluorescence measurement	≈93%

[43] Chewing surfaces feature pits and fissures and approximately 30–40% of such fissures which appear to be intact are carious. This especially applies for children and adolescents.

[44] Both the laser light source and the detection unit are integrated in a handy laser probe which is usually connected to a basic device by optical fibres.

[45] Electrical caries monitoring (ECM) is a comparative measurement technique which is based on the measurement of the electrical resistance of teeth. Since caries features high electrical conductivity in comparison to dentine, lower electrical resistances than the electrical rsistance of dentine indicate the presence of caries.

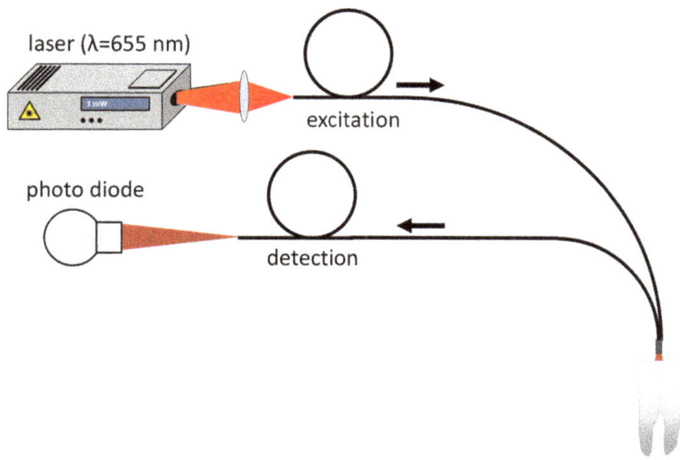

Figure 4.37. Principle of early recognition of caries via laser-induced fluorescence (adapted from [21]).

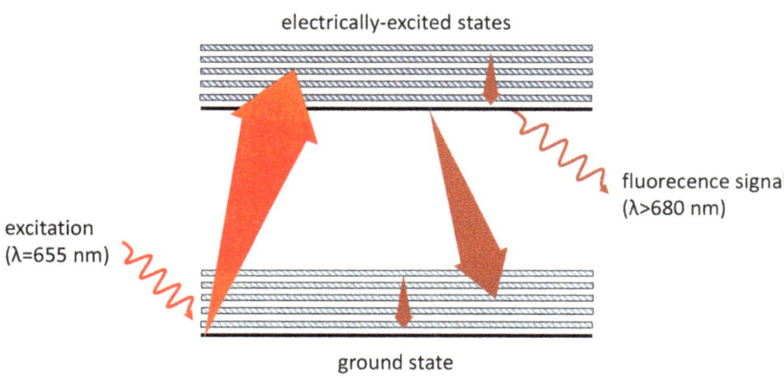

Figure 4.38. Visualisation of the formation of fluorescence during early recognition of caries (adapted from [22]).

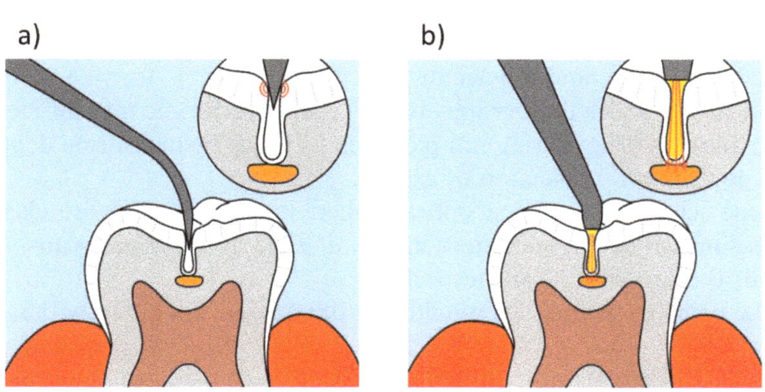

Figure 4.39. Visualisation of the difference in information depth of mechanical probes (a) and laser irradiation (b) during the detection of caries at the bottom of a fissure.

4.11 Lasers in diagnosis—the bottom line

- Spectroscopic measurement techniques allow the wavelength-resolved analysis of material characteristics.
- The principle of excitation spectroscopy is the indirect measurement of discrete absorption bands via the detection of laser-induced fluorescence which corresponds to these absorption bands.
- Infrared spectroscopy is a method of molecular spectroscopy for the identification and quantitative detection of molecules by light-induced excitation of different energy states of molecules.
- The interaction of infrared light and molecules can be classified into three main categories: harmonics of the mid infrared range and combination vibrations, vibrations of covalent bonded electrons of molecules, and general molecular vibrations such as symmetrical and asymmetrical stretching, bending, rocking, wagging and twisting.
- A spectrometer basically consists of a broadband light source, a monochromator and a detector.
- The separation of broadband light into its spectral components can be realised by dispersive refractive elements and diffractive ones which are also referred to as monochromators.
- A special type of infrared spectrometer commonly used in medical analysis is the Fourier-transform infrared (FTIR) spectrometer where the spectrum is determined by interferometric measurements.
- FTIR spectrometers stand out due to short testing times and an improved signal-to-noise ratio.
- Confocal laser scanning microscopes allow the measurement of thin slices, e.g. tissue layers, at a high depth resolution.
- The approach of stimulated emission depletion (STED) microscopy allows the detection of single cells by overcoming the physical limit of resolution of classical microscopes which follows from diffraction.
- Wave front sensing for the detection of defective vision is performed by Shack–Hartmann wave front sensors.
- A Shack–Hartmann wave front sensor basically consists of a laser source, a micro lens array and a detector.
- Optical coherence tomography (OCT) is applied for the interior measurement and analysis of scattering samples such as tissue by measuring depth profiles, e.g. for the early detection of cancer.
- Tissue scans obtained via optical coherence tomography are classified into one-dimensional, two-dimensional and three-dimensional scans, named A-scan, B-scan and C-scan, respectively.
- Pulse oximetry is used for monitoring the oxygen saturation within blood and tissue.
- A pulse oximeter basically consists of a diode laser as light source and a couple of photodetectors, arranged oppositely in a finger clip.

- Synthetic aperture linking (SAL) is a laser-based method for the early diagnosis of rheumatic arthritis.
- The partial pressure and concentration of carbon dioxide within a patient's exhalation air can be measured via optical capnography.
- The laser-induced photoactivation of hematoporphyrin derivative (HpD) is a photodynamic method which allows the diagnosis of tumours and even the devitalisation of tumour cells.
- Flow cytometry is a technique for the differentiation of particles or cells and the analysis of the physical and molecular properties of intact cells on the basis of fluorescence.
- Fluorescence measurements are suitable and powerful methods for early recognition of caries.

References

[1] Arnolds R Einführung in die optischen Grundlagen der IR-Spekroskopie http://www.ir-spektroskopie.de/spec/basics/#3 accessed: 2018-05-02

[2] Siesler H W, Ozaki Y, Kawata S and Heise H M 2008 *Near-infrared Spectroscopy: Principles, Instruments, Applications* (New York: Wiley)

[3] Wildanger D, Patton B R, Schill H, Marseglia L, Hadden J, Knauer S, Schönle A, Rarity J G, O'Brien J L and Hell S W *et al* 2012 *Adv. Mater.* **24** OP309–OP313

[4] Gorlitz F, Hoyer P, Falk H, Kastrup L, Engelhardt J and Hell S W 2014 *Prog. Electromagn. Res.* **147** 57–68

[5] Klar T A, Jakobs S, Dyba M, Egner A and Hell S W 2000 *Proc. Natl. Acad. Sci.* **97** 8206–10

[6] Moneron G and Hell S W 2009 *Opt. Express* **17** 14567–73

[7] Kunzmann M, Schäfer B and Mann K 2005 *Photonik* **1** 52–5

[8] Thews G, Mutschler E and Vaupel P 1991 *Anatomie, Physiologie, Pathophysiologie des Menschen* 1st edn (Stuttgart: Wissenschaftliche Verlagsgesellschaft) ISBN 978-3804723429

[9] Boers M 1995 *J. Rheumatol.* **22** 1783–6

[10] Mulherin D, Fitzgerald O and Bresnihan B 1996 *Rheumatology* **35** 1263–8

[11] Prapavat V 1997 *Anwendung der experimentellen Systemanalyse zur Informationsgewinnung aus Streulicht im Frühstadium entzündlich-rheumatischer Veränderungen* (ecomed)

[12] Prapavat V, Runge W, Mans J, Krause A, Beuthan J and Müller G 1997 *Biomed. Tech./ Biomed. Eng.* **42** 319–26

[13] Berlien H P and Müller G 2000 *Angewandte Lasermedizin - Lehr und Handbuch für Praxis und Klinik* 3rd ed (Berlin: Laser- und Medizin-Technologie) ISBN 3-609-70510-8

[14] Lund P, Heikal A, Maricic M, Krupinski E and Williams C 1995 *Skelet. Radiol.* **24** 591–6

[15] Moan J and Christensen T 1981 *Cancer Lett.* **11** 209–14

[16] Berns M W, Dahlman A, Johnson F M, Burns R, Sperling D, Guiltinan M, Siemens A, Walter R, Wright W and Hammer-Wilson M *et al* 1982 *Cancer Res.* **42** 2325–9

[17] Niemz M H 2013 *Laser-tissue Interactions: Fundamentals and Applications* (Berlin: Springer)

[18] Tegos G, Dai T, Fuchs B B, Coleman J J, Prates R A, Astrakas C St, Denis T G, Ribeiro M S, Mylonakis E and Hamblin M R 2012 *Front. Microbiol.* **3** 120

[19] Brown M and Wittwer C 2000 *Clin. Chem.* **46** 1221–9

[20] Attrill D and Ashley P 2001 *Br. Dent. J.* **190** 440

[21] Lussi A, Hibst R and Paulus R 2004 *J. Dent. Res.* **83** 80–3

[22] Hibst R and Gall R 1998 *Caries Res.* **32** 294

IOP Publishing

Lasers in Medical Diagnosis and Therapy
Basics, applications and future prospects
Stephan Wieneke and Christoph Gerhard

Chapter 5

Lasers in medical therapy

This Chapter provides a short overview on selected established and novel laser-based approaches and methods for the therapy of widespread diseases in orthopaedics, urology, ophthalmology, oncology, cardiology, surgery, and dermatology. For instance, the methods of percutaneous laser disk decompression, laser-induced shock wave lithotripsy, laser-assisted in situ keratomileusis, excimer laser-assisted non-occlusive anastomosis, transmyocardial laser revascularisation and finally the cutting and treatment of bones and tissue are presented. In addition to these methods, the particular diseases to be treated are shortly introduced.

5.1 Lasers in orthopaedics

5.1.1 Intervertebral discs and disc lesions

The human spinal column basically consists of the osseous vertebrae and the intervertebral discs which roughly make a fourth of the entire length of the spinal column. The intervertebral discs act as fibrocartilaginous joints and are composed of a gelatinous core, the nucleus pulposus which mainly consists of water (90%), and a surrounding ring-shaped fibrocartilage, the anulus fibrosus. The supply of the intervertebral discs with vitally important minerals and liquids is not an active, but a passive process based on the penetration of such substances due to a gradient in concentration[1]. In the course of a day, a considerable loss of water occurs in intervertebral discs[2] which is compensated during sleep. However, the underlying swelling power of the discs declines in the course of life. This may lead to different disc lesions, for example disc protrusion. Continuing disc protrusion can

[1] This passive process starts in early infancy. Until the age of two years, the intervertebral discs are supported directly by vasculature.

[2] As a result of this loss of water, the body height of an adult is reduced by approximately 3 cm in the evening with respect to the morning.

doi:10.1088/978-0-7503-1275-2ch5

furthermore be followed by subsequent rupture of the fibrocartilage and leakage of the gelatinous core, which is referred to as spinal disc herniation or prolapsus nuclei pulposi. Another type of disc lesion is the so-called sequestration where material segregates from the disc and accumulates at a certain distance where it can even cause radiculitis. Disc lesions are usually accompanied with violent pain since decayed intervertebral discs impact the involved nerve fibres. In the case of spinal disc herniation, the gelatinous core is replaced towards nerve roots or the spinal canal from where pain is directed to the brain, activating the pain memory. Such diseases or lesions are widespread and have a severe impact on the working capacity, the motivity and the quality of an individal's life. However, classical surgical intervention to the spinal column bears several risks. Against this background, laser-based processes such as percutaneous laser disk decompression are of great interest.

5.1.2 Percutaneous laser disk decompression

The treatment of disc lesions via micro lasers is referred to as percutaneous laser disk decompression (PLDD) [1–3]. Here, the laser light is brought directly to the affected intervertebral disc via an optical fibre which is embedded in a hollow needle. When irradiating the gelatinous core with focussed laser irradiation, a certain volume is vaporised, as shown in figure 5.1, resulting in the removal of core material and a decrease in pressure.

Owing to the ability to deliver a precise dosage of laser irradiation and the accompanying induced effects such as vaporisation and coagulation of intervertebral disc tissue, this special micro laser therapy method allows the treatment of discs of the cervical spine and the lumbar spine which are difficult to access. The therapeutic effects achieved by percutaneous laser disk decompression are (i) the shrinking of the gelatinous core and the accompanying relief of pain, (ii) the inactivation of algesic nerve structures, (iii) the laser-induced inhibition of the formation of neurotransmitters which transfer pain, and (iv) a partial closing of smaller tears at intervertebral discs.

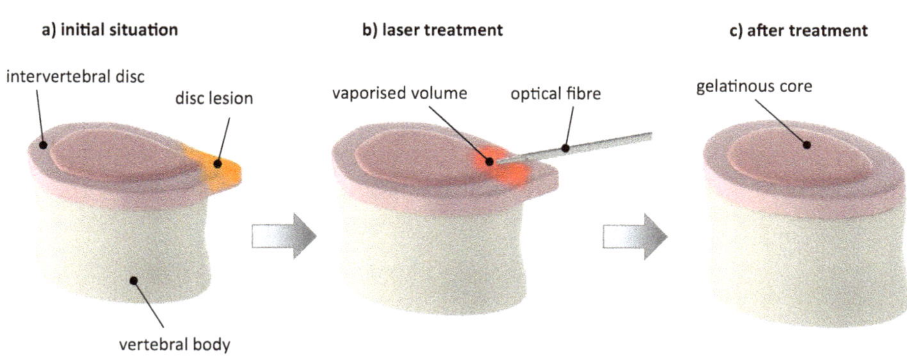

Figure 5.1. Principle of percutaneous laser disk decompression; an intervertebral disc with a lesion (a) is treated by laser irradiation in order to vaporise excess material from the gelatinous core (b), finally leading to a remission of the lesion (c).

Laser parameters applied for percutaneous laser disk decompression (PLDD) [4]

- Laser system: diode laser.
- Wavelength: 980 nm.
- Laser power: 1–10 W.
- Operation mode: continuous wave and pulsed.
- Laser focus diameter: 200 μm.
- Number of fibres: 1.
- Length of catheter system: 40–70 cm.

5.2 Lasers in urology

5.2.1 Kidney stones and nephrolithiasis

Nephrolithiasis is a disease prevalent in adults and is twice as common in men as in women. The kidney stones which cause this disease are formed by the crystallisation of substances which are usually in solution within urine. The mechanisms causing such crystallisation are quite complex and not yet fully understood. However, different causes which might interact in some cases can be identified:

- Dehydration due to insufficient drinking, exudation, or diarrhoea, leading to an increase in a concentration of substances which can crystallise
- Poor or wrong nutrition[3] (e.g. mainly consisting of either milk and dairy products or food rich in protein), giving rise to an excess of calcium in urine or purine in blood; this may lead to an increased uric acid concentration, followed by lithiasis
- Immobilisation, e.g. of bedfast patients, causing the depletion of calcium from bones which accumulates in the urine
- Urinary tract infections
- Metabolic diseases.

The formed kidney stones occur either directly within the kidney or within the urinary tract collection system. The size of such stones ranges from a few millimetres to several centimetres[4]. The symptoms of nephrolithiasis strongly depend on the size, position and mobility of the kidney stones. In severe cases, renal colic can occur which is accompanied with violent pain in the back and the lower abdomen. Nephrolithiasis is often detected accidentally during ultrasonic or radiological examination. In some cases, smaller kidney stones are excreted during micturition. However, such spontaneous excretion fails to appear in many cases and lithotripsy becomes necessary. This can be performed in different ways such as for example via extracorporeal shock wave therapy (ESWT) or laser-induced shock wave lithotripsy (LISL).

[3] For instance, several esculents such as spinach or green tea contain an increased portion of oxalic acid. This acid forms calcium oxalate stones by oxalo-calcic lithiasis.

[4] A kidney stone with a size of several centimetres is the so-called staghorn calculus which can even fill the entire renal pelvis.

5.2.2 Laser-induced shock wave lithotripsy

As presented in more detail in section 3.2.4, high laser intensity and low laser pulse durations result in photo-disruption in tissue and the formation of plasma. The latter is due to optical breakdown within the laser focus and is accompanied with the formation of shock waves. This effect is applied for laser-induced fragmentation of kidney stones via LISL [5]. Here, flash lamp-pumped dye lasers, alexandrite lasers, and Q-switched Nd:YAG lasers with pulse durations in the range from 10 ns to 2 μs and pulse energies of about 50–100 mJ are used [6]. The laser is focussed in the vicinity of the particular stone and a plasma is ignited. The resulting shock wave can exhibit an extreme pressure value (several 100 bar) and thus induce the fragmentation of the stone. In order to induce this effect, the laser light has to be brought into the human body which is realised by optical fibres[5]. For focussing, the fibre end is either shaped spherically or equipped with a micro-optical imaging system. It should be noted that the shock wave selectively affects the stone, whereas its impact on the neighbouring tissue is negligible. Finally, the method of LISL can also be applied for the fragmentation of other intracorporal stones, i.e. bladder stones or gall stones. In the latter case, the novel approach of LISL using frequency-doubled double-pulse Nd: YAG (FREDDY) lasers has turned out to be a promising technique for the selective removal of difficult choledocholithiasis, also known as bile duct stones. As shown in figure 5.2, two laser pulses of different wavelengths are applied. These pulses cross the tissue, but are absorbed by stones and induce fragmentation [7–9]. A laser setup as used for this approach is shown in figure 5.3.

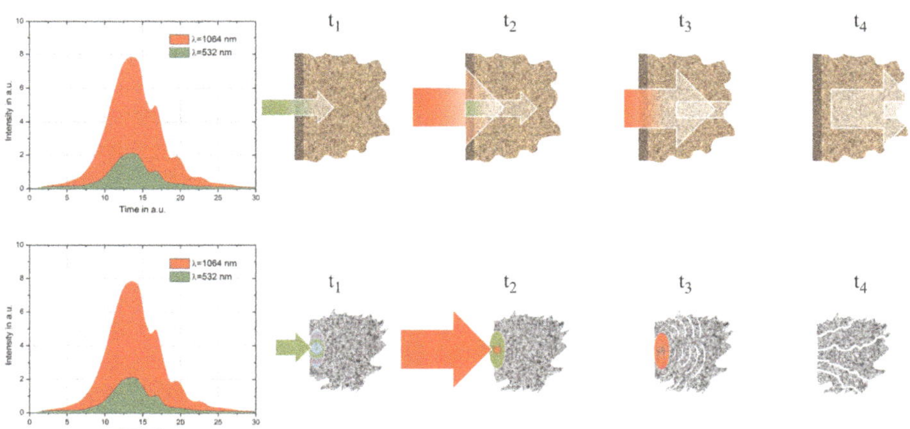

Figure 5.2. Impact of double pulses on tissue (top) and stone (bottom) at different points in time t where $t_4 > t_3 > t_2 > t_1$. The laser light is not absorbed by the tissue (top), but by the stones (bottom) where two temporally-shifted shock waves are induced, causing the efficient fragmentation of stones.

[5] The fibres used here are embedded in a flexible endoscope which contains additional fibres for illumination and observation and features a maximum outer diameter of 1.9 mm.

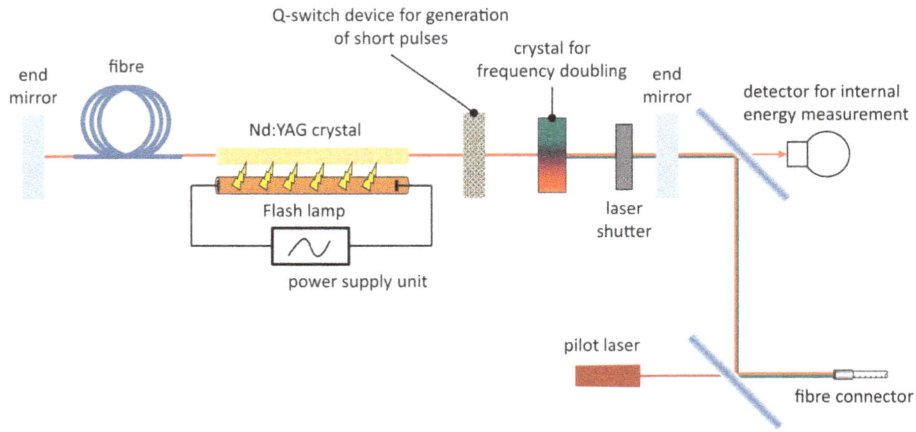

Figure 5.3. Setup of a frequency-doubled double-pulse Nd:YAG laser setup for LISL (adapted from [9]).

Typical laser parameters applied for LISL

- Laser system: Nd:YAG laser or Ho:YAG laser.
- Wavelength: 1064 nm or 2080 nm (partially λ = 2123 nm).
- Laser pulse peak power: up to 15 kW.
- Laser pulse energy: 50 mJ up to 500 mJ.
- Operation mode: pulsed (pulse duration 5 ns–150 μs).
- Laser focus diameter: 120 μm.

5.3 Lasers in ophthalmology

5.3.1 Structure and properties of the human eye

The combination of the eyes and the brain represents the archetype of any imaging system invented by man and the human eye could be referred to as the masterpiece of evolution. Its basic setup is shown in figure 5.4 and its most important optical properties are listed in table 5.1.

The optical power of the human eye principally results from the curvature of the cornea with a typical radius of curvature of 5.6 mm and from the difference in index of refraction of the cornea and the surrounding air of approximately Δn = 0.37. Dynamic focussing, the so-called accommodation of the eye, is realised by the eye lens which is either contracted or relaxed by the ciliary muscle, resulting in a change in surface shape and focal length, respectively. This allows clear and sharp imaging of objects at a minimum distance of approximately 15 cm. However, the standardised distance of most distinct vision which is used for the calculation of imaging optical systems is specified to be 25 cm by default. The capability of an eye of focussing incoming light is referred to as optical power. In ophthalmology, the unit of this value is the dioptre, abbreviated dpt. The dioptric value p of a human eye is given by the reciprocal value of a metre as the basic unit and is calculated according to

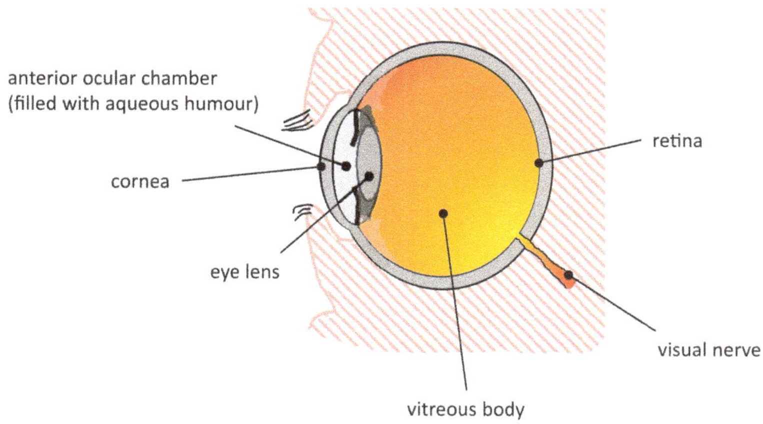

Figure 5.4. Basic setup of the human eye including all essential components required for imaging.

Table 5.1. Selection of the most important optical properties of the human eye.

	Indices of refraction
Component	**Value**
Vitreous body	1.336
Aqueous humour	1.336
Cornea	1.368
Eye lens	1.37–1.42
	Focal lengths and distances
Parameter	**Value**
Front focal length (in air)	14–17 mm
Back focal length (within the eye ball)	19–23 mm
Distance of most distinct vision	150 mm–∞
Standardised distance of most distinct vision S_0	250 mm
	Geometry and sensitivity
Parameter	**Value**
Pupil diameter	1–8 mm
Resolution power (at S_0)	10 μm
Retina sensitivity	1.5×10^{-17} W per photoreceptor (≈ 30 photons per second)
Maximum of spectral sensitivity (at daylight)	555 nm

$$p = \frac{1}{f} \tag{5.1}$$

with f being the eye's focal length[6], given in metres[7]. The measurement of the focal length of any eye thus allows its defective vision to be determined, which is specified

[6] For instance, a dioptric value of $p = 5$ corresponds to a focal length of $f = 0.2$ m.
[7] In physics, the focal length is usually given in millimetres if not otherwise specified.

with respect to the sight of a healthy eye. It is thus either a positive or negative value. In normal cases, the optical power amounts to approximately 43 dpt for the cornea and to about 19 dpt for the eye lens. The optical power of an emmetropic eye is 65 dpt, which is not only the sum of the two above-mentioned optical powers since the anterior ocular chamber and the vitreous body have to be taken into account additionally. A long-sighted (hyperopic) eye, see figure 5.5(a), exhibits a positive dioptric value, its optical power is thus lower than the reference value. This means that the focal length of the focussing elements of such an eye is too long and incoming light is focussed to a plane behind the retina and the fovea centralis, respectively. In contrast, the focal point of a short-sighted (myopic) eye which is denoted by a negative dioptric value is found within the vitreous body before the retina, as shown in figure 5.5(b).

Defective vision can have several, partially interacting reasons such as a corneal irregularity or a deformation of the entire eye ball. This restriction can be reduced by the use of lasers. In this case, far-sightedness (hyperopia) and short-sightedness (myopia) and even non-rotational defects and aberrations such as astigmatism are not corrected indirectly by introducing a further, correcting optical element such as glasses or contact lenses to the eye, but directly via a selective re-shaping of the cornea as shown in figure 5.5(c) and presented in the following two sections.

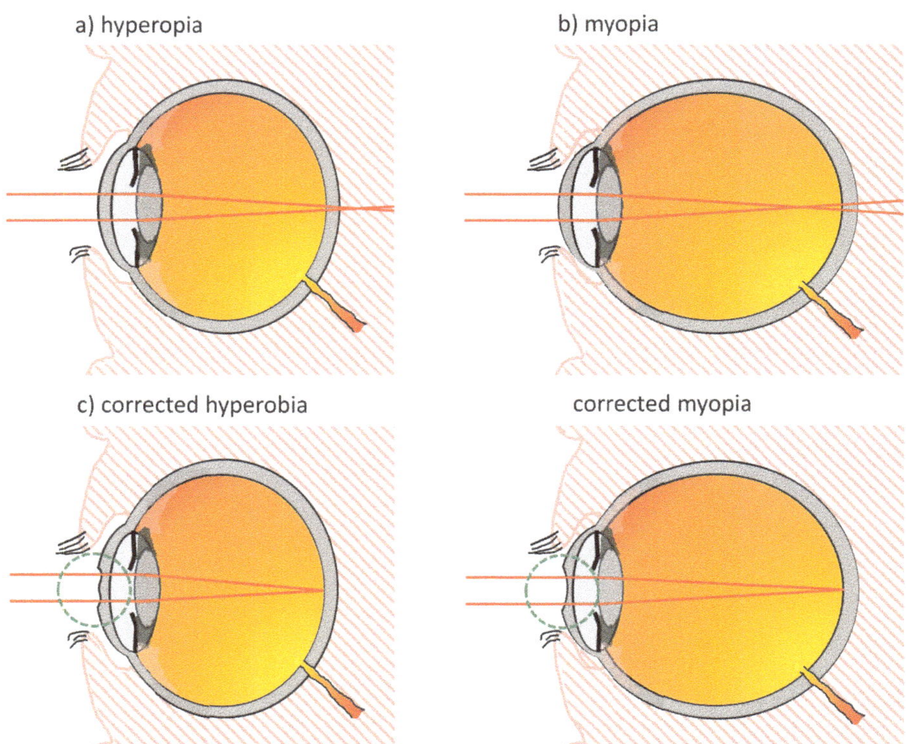

Figure 5.5. Beam path in a long-sighted (a) and a short-sighted (b) eye including the beam path of the particular eye after correction of defective vision by re-shaping of the cornea (c).

5.3.2 Classical laser-assisted *in situ* keratomileusis

In general, the term keratomileusis describes the surgical correction of defective vision via re-shaping the cornea. When performed with the aid of laser irradiation, this intervention is referred to as laser-assisted *in situ* keratomileusis (LASIK). This method consists of several subsequent steps, as shown in figure 5.6, where the essential steps are the suction process, the preparation of the cornea, the actual laser-based re-shaping of the cornea and the final wound closure.

In order to fix the eye and to prevent its movement during the application of laser light, a suction ring is placed on the eye (figure 5.6(a)). In the course of the following preparation of the cornea, a thin slice of cornea, the so-called flap, with a thickness of approximately 180 μm is cut with the aid of a precision dissecting knife (figure 5.6(b)). This slice is not fully cut off, but hinged away and the interior of the cornea is uncovered (figure 5.6(c)). The actual re-shaping of the cornea is performed after these initial steps. It is carried out with the aid of focussed laser irradiation provided by an argon fluoride excimer laser. For the correction of far-sightedness, a ring-shaped area around the centre of the cornea is removed, whereas the removal of the cornea centre is required for the correction of short-sightedness (figure 5.6(d)). In the course of this process, eventual corneal irregularity is corrected simultaneously by shaping a spherical surface. The thickness t of the cornea material to be removed, i.e. the ablation depth (given in μm), is given by the Munnerlyn equation according to [10]

$$t = z^2 \cdot \frac{p}{3}. \tag{5.2}$$

Here, z is the diameter of the zone where material is removed (given in mm) and p is the ametropia to be corrected (given in dpt). The maximum ablation depth of approximately 160–300 μm is limited by the thickness of the cornea. When exceeding the given limit of a residual layer of approximately 250 μm which should remain underneath the flap in order to ensure the stability of the cornea, the residual

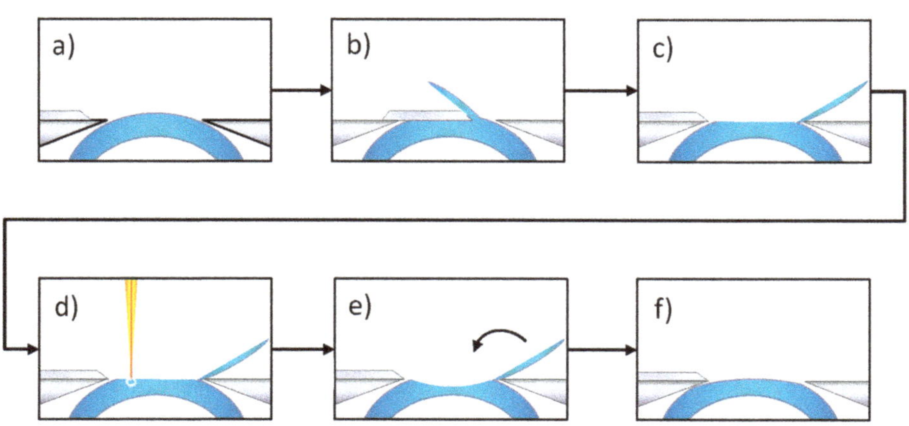

Figure 5.6. Procedure of classical laser-assisted *in situ* keratomileusis; a detailed description of the single steps (a)–(f) is given in the text.

cornea thickness becomes critical[8]. The zone affected by LASIK where the cornea material is removed exhibits a diameter of approximately 6 mm; it corresponds to the pupil diameter at least. The thickness of the flap is 180 μm as mentioned above. For instance, a cornea layer with a thickness of 120 μm has to be removed in order to correct an ametropia of 10 dpt according to equation (5.2). Prior to a LASIK operation, the thickness of the cornea thus has to amount to 120 μm (material to be removed) + 180 μm (flap thickness) + 250 μm (residual cornea layer) = 550 μm. Once the re-shaping of the cornea is finished, the flap is finally placed on the laser-ablated cornea surface (figure 5.6(e)) and acts as a body's own plaster which is fixed by adhesive power (figure 5.6(f)). As mentioned above, argon fluoride (ArF) excimer lasers with an emission wavelength of 193 nm are applied for LASIK. This is due to the fact that the cornea exhibits high absorbance for this wavelength and the incoming laser irradiation is thus efficiently absorbed within a thin near-surface layer. The neighbouring tissue is consequently not affected. For ArF excimer laser irradiation, the laser ablation threshold fluence of cornea amounts to approximately 50 mJ cm^{-2}. At higher fluences, the ablation depth increases logarithmically, which can be explained by the blow-off model (see section 3.2.3). According to the Beer–Lambert law, the laser fluence F within tissue decreases exponentially as expressed by

$$F = F_0 \cdot e^{-x/x_{\mathrm{opt}}} \tag{5.3}$$

where F_0 is the initial maximum fluence required for initiating ablation, x is the position and x_{opt} is the depth of penetration of laser light into the tissue[9]. Up to the depth where the fluence has reached the value of the ablation threshold F_{th}, the tissue is photo-ablated (see figure 3.32). The ablation depth x_{abl} can thus be written as

$$x_{\mathrm{abl}} = x_{\mathrm{opt}} \cdot \ln\left(\frac{F_{\mathrm{th}}}{F_0}\right). \tag{5.4}$$

This demonstrates the above-mentioned logarithmic interrelationship of the ablation depth and the fluence, as also shown in figure 5.7.

In clinical practice, laser-assisted *in situ* keratomileusis is performed at laser fluences in the range from 100 mJ cm^{-2} to 250 mJ cm^{-2}. According to equation (5.4), the corresponding ablation depths are approximately 100–500 nm per laser pulse.

5.3.3 Femto-laser-assisted *in situ* keratomileusis

Classical LASIK, as described above, is based on the high absorption of the cornea for the excimer laser wavelength used. However, ablation can generally also be obtained at wavelengths where the cornea features high transmittance. In this case, the ablation process is based on a completely different underlying mechanism, i.e. nonlinear effects induced by extremely high laser intensity (see section 3.2.4). Such

[8] Special attention should be paid to this issue since insufficient residual cornea thickness can result in an iatrogenic keratectasia.

[9] The optical depth of penetration of argon fluoride (ArF) excimer laser light into the cornea amounts to approximately 330 nm.

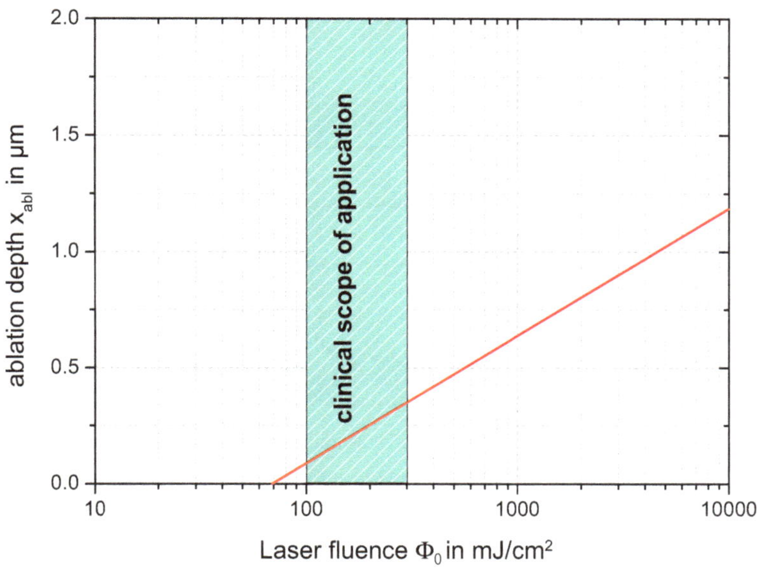

Figure 5.7. Ablation depth of cornea versus laser fluence. The ablation threshold is found at a value of approximately 50 mJ cm^{-2} (adapted from [11]).

high intensities preferentially occur for focussed ultra-short laser pulses with pulse durations in the femtosecond range. It should be noted that the extraordinarily high intensities are only found in the focal area with a dimension of some microns. This allows focussing light into deeper regions of a transparent medium where material modification or cutting of material selectively occurs within the focal area, but not on the material's surface. In this way structures within bulk material can be generated without any damage of the front or back face of the transparent medium. When applying this technique to laser-based refractive surgery in ophthalmology, it is referred to as femto-LASIK or fs-LASIK. The different steps of this method are summarised in figure 5.8.

It turns out that in contrast to classical LASIK, no flap preparation by mechanical cutting is required [12, 14]. The incoming laser beam is focussed into the cornea and an internal cut, i.e. the lower edge of the material to be removed, is ablated by photo-disruption (figure 5.8(a)). Subsequently, the upper edge is produced (figure 5.8(b)), resulting in the formation of a meniscus-shaped slice, the lenticule (figure 5.8(c))[10]. Finally, a gap with a thickness of approximately 2–3 mm is cut (figure 5.8(d)) and the lenticule is removed with the aid of a micro gripper (figure 5.8(e)). Due to adhesive power, the remaining gap within the cornea is closed (figure 5.8(f)). Depending on the shape of the meniscus removed in the course of this process, the refractive power of the eye is finally corrected.

[10] Based on the shape of the laser-cut slice, this technique is called small incision lenticule extraction (SMILE).

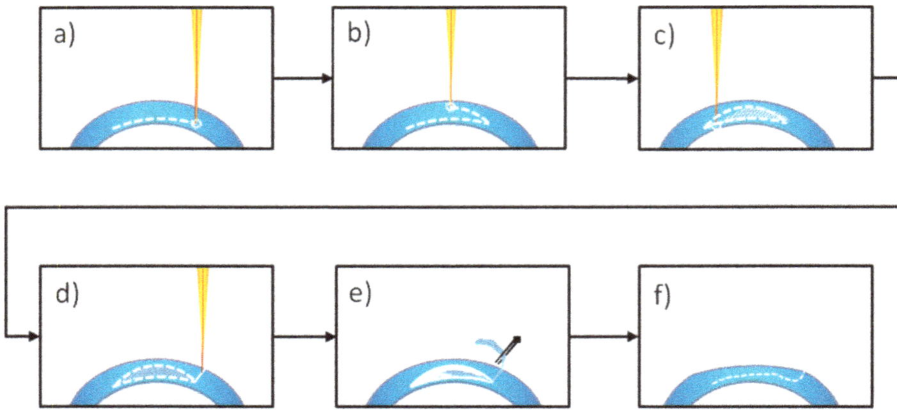

Figure 5.8. Procedure of femto-laser-assisted *in situ* keratomileusis; a detailed description of the single steps (a)–(f) is given in the text (adapted from [12, 13]).

Typical laser parameters applied for classical laser-assisted *in situ* keratomileusis (LASIK)

- Laser system: excimer laser.
- Wavelength: typically ArF $\lambda = 193$ nm.
- Laser pulse peak power: up to 15 kW.
- Fluence: up to 250 mJ cm^{-2}.
- Pulse duration: typically 10–20 ns.
- Pulse repetition rate: up to 20 Hz.
- Laser focus diameter: about 900 μm (Gaussian beam profile).

5.3.4 Laser treatment of retinal vascular disorders

Generally, eye diseases affecting the retinal blood vessels are referred to as retinal vascular disorders. Such diseases may result from high blood pressure which can cause a narrowing, hardening or even leaking of blood vessels as well as arteriosclerosis, i.e. the swelling of artery walls. Retinal vascular diseases can be classified into different sub-categories such as hypertensive retinopathy, central retinal artery occlusion (CRAO), and retinal vein occlusion (RVO) which can be segmented into branch retinal vein occlusion (BRVO) on the one hand and central retinal vein occlusion (CRVO) on the other hand. Both types of RVO can cause macular oedema and neovascularisation. Moreover, diabetic retinopathy is a widespread eye disease[11] where the retina is damaged due to microangiopathy, i.e. the damage of small blood vessels, induced by diabetes mellitus. For the treatment of the above-mentioned different types of retinal vein occlusion and diabetic retinopathy, three different laser treatment methods based on the effect of laser-induced coagulation have been developed: focal

[11] Diabetic retinopathy affects approximately 80% of people who suffered from diabetes for at least 20 years.

treatment, grid treatment, and panretinal treatment. Here, laser irradiation is focussed onto the retina in order to induce photocoagulation as shown in 5.9.

Focal treatment is applied in order to seal leaking blood vessels of patients with diabetic retinopathy locally. For this purpose, such leaking vessels are identified and located (e.g. via angiography) and selectively irradiated by focussed laser irradiation as shown in figure 5.9(left) in order to induce coagulation and thus to reduce leakage of liquid. This approach is normally used for treating proliferative diabetic retinopathy at its early stage. Another method is the so-called grid treatment which is applied in the case of diffuse leakage of vessels. As shown in figure 5.9(middle), small laser burns are realised at low laser intensity around the macula lutea in a locally selective manner. The area or grid to be treated is usually identified via optical coherence tomography, see section 4.4, or fluorescein angiography. This approach is suitable for the treatment of macular oedema caused by diabetes mellitus or vessel blockages. Finally, panretinal treatment[12] allows the reduction of the oxygen demand of the retina and consequently the area of ischemic retinal tissue. This is realised by creating approximately 1600–2000 laser burns which are arranged concentrically around the fovea centralis and the optic nerve, see figure 5.9(right). It is applied for the treatment of productive diabetic retinopathy and reduces the risk

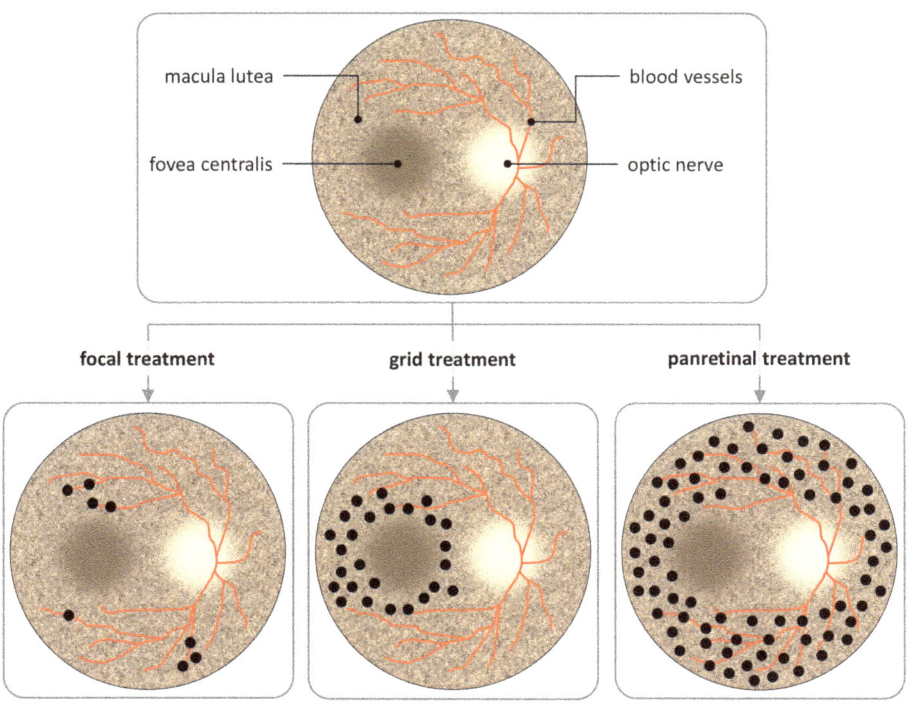

Figure 5.9. The main components of the retina (top) and three different approaches for the laser treatment of retinal vascular disorders (bottom) by punctual laser-induced photocoagulation (black spots).

[12] This type of treatment is also referred to as scatter laser treatment.

of neovascularisation and potentially accompanying hemorrhaging and oedemas by destroying abnormal blood vessels[13]. Panretinal treatment has to be performed in several sessions and should eventually be repeated regularly since proliferative diabetic retinopathy may cause new bleedings or even glaucoma.

5.4 Lasers in oncology

In oncology, lasers are applied for the treatment of malignant and benign tumours via the minimal-invasive method of laser-induced thermotherapy (LITT). Here, diode laser or Nd:YAG laser irradiation at a wavelength in the range 800–1064 nm and a typical power of 5–25 W is brought to the affected tissue (e.g. liver, brain, or prostate) with the aid of an optical fibre[14]. This fibre is equipped with an angled, spherically-shaped or plane fibre tip (see section 2.3.1) or other special diffuser tip applicators, as shown in figure 5.10, depending on the volume of tissue to be irradiated.

The laser light is then absorbed in the course of the application which usually lasts for 25 minutes. Due to absorption, the tissue is heated locally up to 45–100 °C, thus inducing interstitial coagulation and further hyperthermia effects. With respect to tumours, it is regarded as assured that a tissue temperature higher than 40.5 °C leads to damage to tumours and has even a cytocidal and inhibitory impact on malignant tissue. Moreover, hypothermia causes overheating of tumour cells which results in an alteration of the tumour's metabolism and an accompanying inhibition in tumour reproduction. Based on the type and state of a tumour, a precise adjustment of the laser parameters (wavelength, power, exposure time etc) and the choice of appropriate equipment, mainly the type and number of fibre tips, becomes necessary for effective treatment. This also applies to the monitoring of the procedure and the induced increase in tissue temperature in order to verify the formation of sufficient hypothermia of the tumour. The basic sequence of LITT is as follows. First, the affected tumorous tissue is examined via magnetic resonance imaging (MRI) with the aid of an intravenous contrast medium. Second, the tumour is punctured in order to generate a channel for the optical fibre and the diffuser tip applicator. This

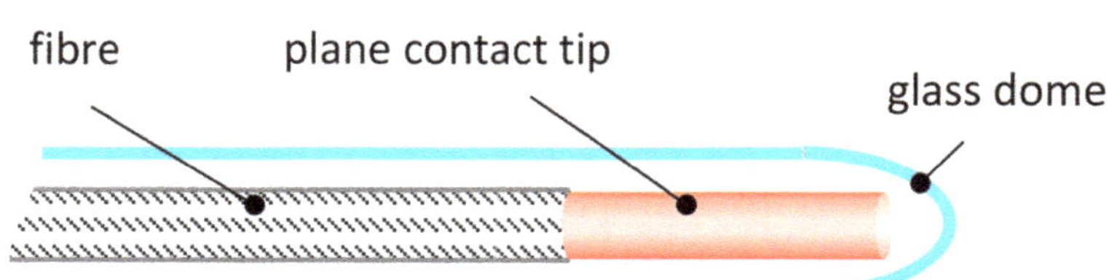

Figure 5.10. Schematic of a diffuser tip applicator as applied for controlled heating of tissue via laser-induced thermotherapy.

---

[13] Panretinal treatment is a powerful method for laser treatment of retinal vascular disorders and allows the risk of severe vision loss to be reduced by 50% [15].

[14] Where possible, LITT is an ambulant transdermal administration but it can also be applied in the course of surgical intervention.

intervention is controlled via ultrasonic monitoring or computed tomography (CT) scans. Finally, the actual LITT process is started where a catheter is inserted into the generated channel and carries the applicator. In the course of the LITT process, the rise in temperature and the temperature distribution within the irradiated tissue are monitored via MRI. In order to prevent overheating of the applicator, the catheter is equipped with an internal cooling circuit as shown in figure 5.11. Once the application is finished, the result is controlled via MRI and an intravenous contrast medium and the punctured tissue is closed with fibrin sealant.

In order to increase the efficiency of LITT and to reduce the duration of treatment, respectively, the so-called power mode can be applied. Here, the output power of the used continuous wave laser is modulated. As shown in figure 5.12, the therapy starts at comparatively high laser power, which is stepwise reduced in the course of the irradiation.

The goal of this approach is to apply high laser powers at an early stage of the therapy when the diffuser tip applicator used is not heated. Subsequently, the power is reduced in order to compensate the applicator's heating and to control hyperthermic effects within the irradiated tissue. The comparison of the power mode and the continuous mode in terms of contact temperature and damage volume is shown in figure 5.13. It turns out that the contact temperature at the diffuser tip surface reaches its maximum value much faster in the case of power mode application. This leads to faster coagulation and the maximum volume of damaged tissue is obtained after an irradiation time of 300 s. In contrast, it takes twice the time until the maximum damaged tissue volume is reached when working in continuous mode. Further, the volume is much smaller in this case when compared to the volume resulting for LITT in power mode. The latter thus stands out due to efficiency and time saving.

Typical laser parameters applied for LITT

- Laser system: Nd:YAG laser.
- Wavelength: 1064 nm.
- Operation mode: continuous wave or pulsed.

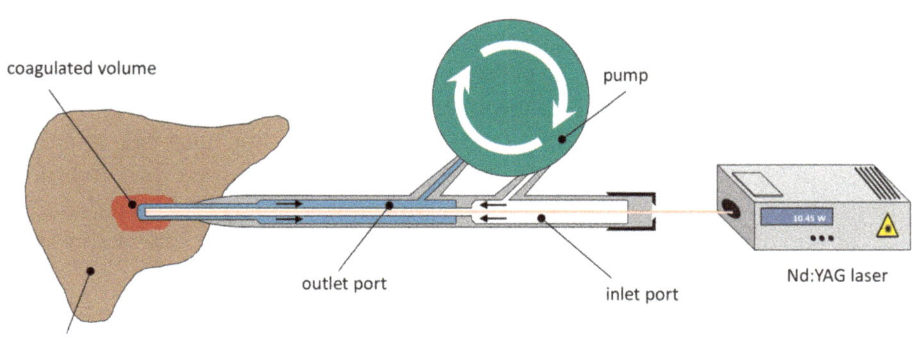

Figure 5.11. Visualisation of laser-induced thermotherapy applying a catheter with internal cooling circuit in order to prevent overheating (adapted from [16]).

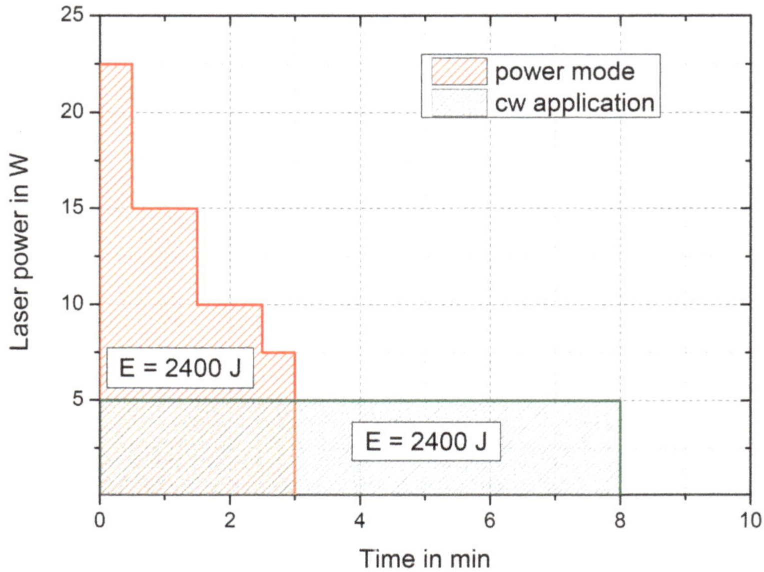

Figure 5.12. Visualisation of the laser power applied to tissue over time during interstitial coagulation by laser-induced thermotherapy in power mode (adapted from [16]).

- Fluence (depends on the used applicator): up to 60 J cm^{-2}.
- Power (depends on the used applicator): up to 60 W.
- Repetition rate: typically 1–20 Hz.
- Laser spot diameter: typically 3–12 mm.

5.5 Lasers in cardiology

5.5.1 Excimer laser-assisted non-occlusive anastomosis

The classical approach for the abatement of symptoms caused by aneurysms, the bypass operation, bears certain risks. In the course of such an operation, the affected artery needs to be blocked as long as the bypass is placed. This procedure may result in an undersupply of oxygen to the brain and even cause apoplexy in severe cases. Aneurysms are thus generally difficult to treat. Basically, an aneurysm is a pathologic local enlargement of an artery or blood vessel[15] which consequently increases the vessel's cross section and thus impacts blood flow. There are different main kinds of aneurysms[16], the true aneurysm (aneurysma verum), the false aneurysm or pseudoaneurysm (aneurisma spurium/falsum), and the aneurysma dissecans which follows from dissection of a vascular wall as shown in figure 5.14.

In order to reduce or even to avoid the risk of undersupply of oxygen to the brain during bypass surgery, a laser-based technique, the excimer laser-assisted

[15] Aneurysms can either be congenital or occur in the course of lifetime.

[16] The most common type of aneurysm is the aortic aneurysm, i.e. a true aneurysm.

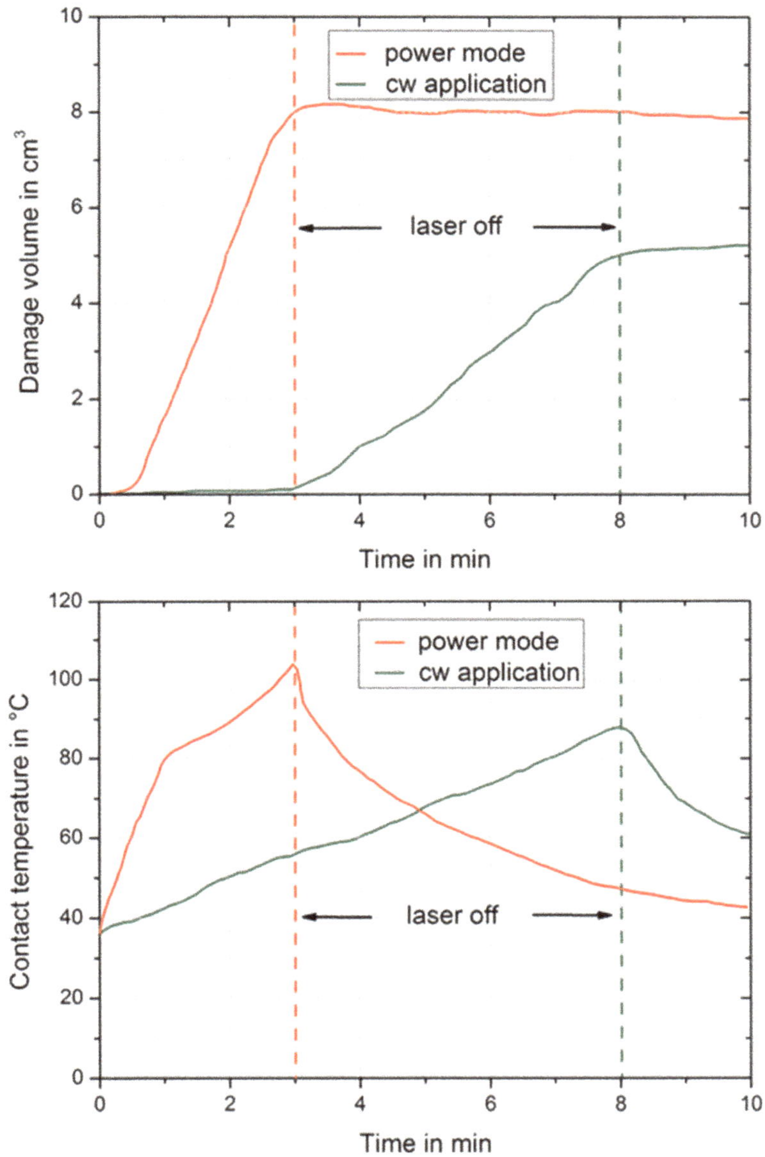

Figure 5.13. Comparison of the damaged volume (top) and the contact temperature (bottom) achieved by laser-induced thermotherapy in power mode and continuous mode (adapted from [17]).

non-occlusive anastomosis (ELANA) was developed and investigated in the last decades [18–20]. This approach allows extracranial-to-intracranial and intracranial-to-intracranial bypass surgery without interrupting the blood supply of the brain. For this purpose, a ring made of platinum with a diameter of 2.6–2.8 mm[17] is sewn on the bypass which is made of donated blood vessels, usually veins from

[17] For distal anastomosis via ELANA, the minimum diameter of the artery is 2.6 mm.

the leg, in a first step as shown in figure 5.15(a). The bypass is then sewn on the artery, see figure 5.15(b), and a circular flap is cut by laser irradiation using a catheter with integrated optical fibre (shown in figure 5.15(c)). Both parts of the bypass are closed with clips in the course of these steps and during sewing of both ends of the donated blood vessel (see figure 5.15(d)) in order to assure blood flow towards the brain via the aneurysm. After the connection between the artery and the bypass is opened (see figure 5.15(e)), the artery is finally pinched in front of and behind the aneurysm, so that the blood exclusively flows through the bypass, as shown in figure 5.15(f).

The catheter used for ELANA normally consists of different optical fibres for laser beam guidance, illumination and monitoring, and an additional tube which is

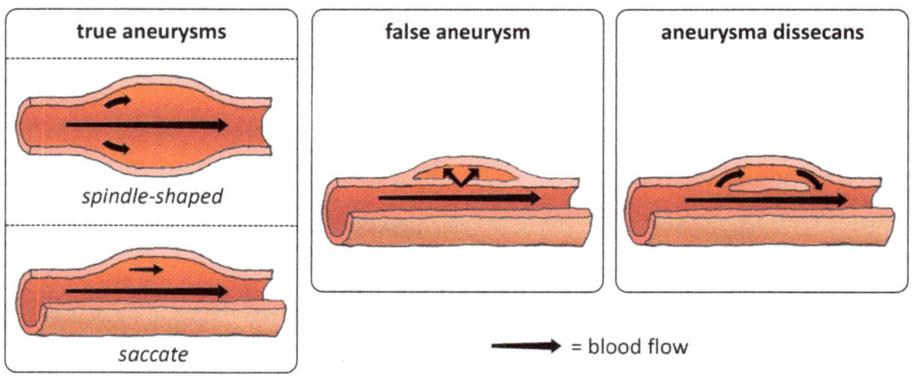

Figure 5.14. Visualisation of the three main types of aneurysms.

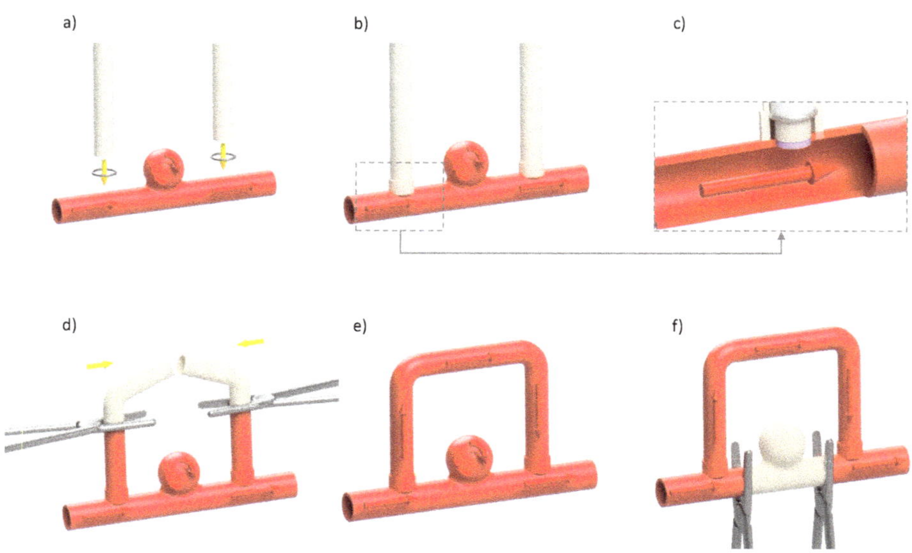

Figure 5.15. Principle of ELANA for the treatment of aneurysms; for a detailed description see the text (adapted from [21]).

connected to an external vacuum pump. This allows the generation of low pressure within the area of interest, leading to the suction of the artery wall onto the used platinum ring which acts as template for precise laser cutting. The end cap of the tube is made of metal and features a certain pattern, the so-called grid. Here, the cut flap is fixed and can be removed from the cutting zone.

Laser parameters applied for ELANA

- Laser system: xenon chloride excimer laser.
- Wavelength: 308 nm.
- Pulse duration: 110–200 ns.
- Pulse energy: 200–300 mJ.
- Pulse repetition rate: 50–200 Hz.
- Laser focus diameter: 60 μm.
- Number of fibres: approximately 180.
- Length of catheter system: 40–70 cm.

5.5.2 Transmyocardial laser revascularisation

Transmyocardial laser revascularisation (TMLR) is a laser-based therapy method applied in the case of severe coronary heart disease [22, 23]. It is used for the treatment of the symptoms of such diseases in order to alleviate the pain of diseased patients. The pain results from a stenosis of the coronary blood vessels, e.g. by calcification, resulting in insufficient perfusion of the heart. Consequently, the patient suffers from angina pectoris and even life-threatening infarct can occur. Classical treatment methods such as stretching[18] the blood vessels or bypass surgery may cause a hardening of the vessels and approximately 20% of the patients report discomfort after such intervention. Against this background, transmyocardial laser revascularisation was developed in recent decades. This method is mainly performed using carbon dioxide lasers with an emission wavelength of 10.6 μm and a pulse duration of 50 ms. As shown in figure 5.16, a number of channels[19] are drilled into the myocardial muscle via laser perforation. For this purpose, the heart has to be exposed, i.e. the thorax has to be opened. This surgical intervention is continuously monitored via transesophageal echocardiogram which is carried out from the oesophagus. As a result of laser-induced perforation, the myocardial muscle becomes efficiently soaked with blood from the heart chambers and new blood vessels are formed starting from the laser-generated channels. Finally, the perfusion of the heart is improved.

The laser is applied at the end of the diastole since at that point in time the heart is filled with blood which absorbs the incoming laser irradiation well. This procedure reduces the risk of inducing damage at the myocardial muscle's surface and the cardiac valves. Once the myocardial muscle is perforated, a laser-induced vapour cloud occurs within the ventricle and is immediately resorbed by the circulation.

[18] The stretching of blood vessels is usually performed by balloon dilatation. This technique is also referred to as percutaneous transluminal coronary angioplasty (PTCA).

[19] I.e. approximately 20 channels with a distance of approximately 1 cm between each other.

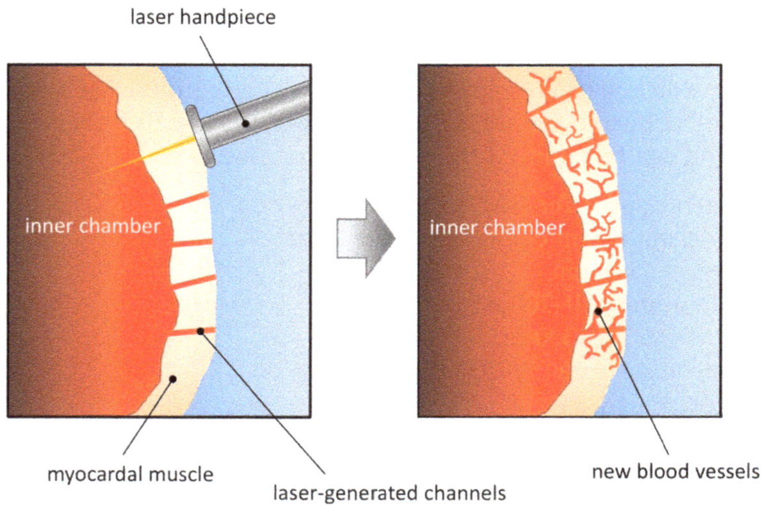

Figure 5.16. Principle of increasing the perfusion of the heart via transmyocardial laser revascularisation (adapted from [24]).

This vapour cloud thus travels through the arterial system and can be detected via echocardiograms, indicating an actually completed channel and thus monitoring the laser perforation process. Bleedings at the surface of the heart normally stop without any styptic intervention or surgical haemostatics. At the end of this surgical intervention, a cardiac stimulator is usually connected to the heart's surface and a thoracic drainage is applied. Finally, the thorax is closed and the operation is finished.

Transmyocardial laser revascularisation can also be performed using holmium lasers at an emission wavelength of 2.06 μm. Here, the main advantage is the possibility of laser light guidance by optical fibres which allows the use of catheters. The heart thus does not need to be exposed by extensive surgical intervention since here, the catheter is inserted into the ventricle and the myocardial muscle is laser-perforated from the inside to the outside. However, the heat affected zone of thermal damage is much higher in the case of holmium laser irradiation with respect to the use of carbon dioxide lasers. This follows from the notable difference in absorption and depth of penetration[20], respectively, of both laser wavelengths by human tissue. Thus, transmyocardial laser revascularisation via carbon dioxide laser irradiation exhibits a number of advantages such as for example the reduction of necrosis. Moreover, the intraventricular use of catheters as applied for holmium laser-based TMLR may cause arrhythmia and traumata of the heart.

Typical laser parameters applied for TMLR

- Laser system: CO_2 laser or Ho:YAG laser.
- Wavelength: 10.6 μm or 2.06 μm.

[20] The depth of penetration of carbon dioxide laser irradiation into tissue amounts to approximately 17 μm, whereas this value is approximately 17 times higher for holmium laser irradiation (290 μm).

- Operation mode: pulsed.
- Energy per pulse: 1–20 J.
- Pulse duration: typically 25–50 ms.
- Power (depends on the used applicator): up to 1000 W.
- Laser spot diameter: typically 1 mm.

5.6 Lasers in surgery

5.6.1 Basics of laser cutting and drilling

During laser cutting or drilling of bones or tissue, the main parameter of interest is the cutting or drilling depth. This depth can be derived from a simplified model as follows. When assuming that the energy required for the vaporisation of a certain unit of volume does not depend on the parameters of the tissue to be ablated, the cutting or drilling depth d should be proportional to the exposure time t and intensity I of laser irradiation as expressed by

$$d^{(x,\,y)} = \int I_t^{(x,\,y)} dt. \tag{5.5}$$

Here, the term $d^{(x,\,y)}$ is the cutting or drilling depth at the position (x, y) of the laser beam profile, as shown in figure 5.17, and $I^{(x,\,y)}$ is the intensity at this position.

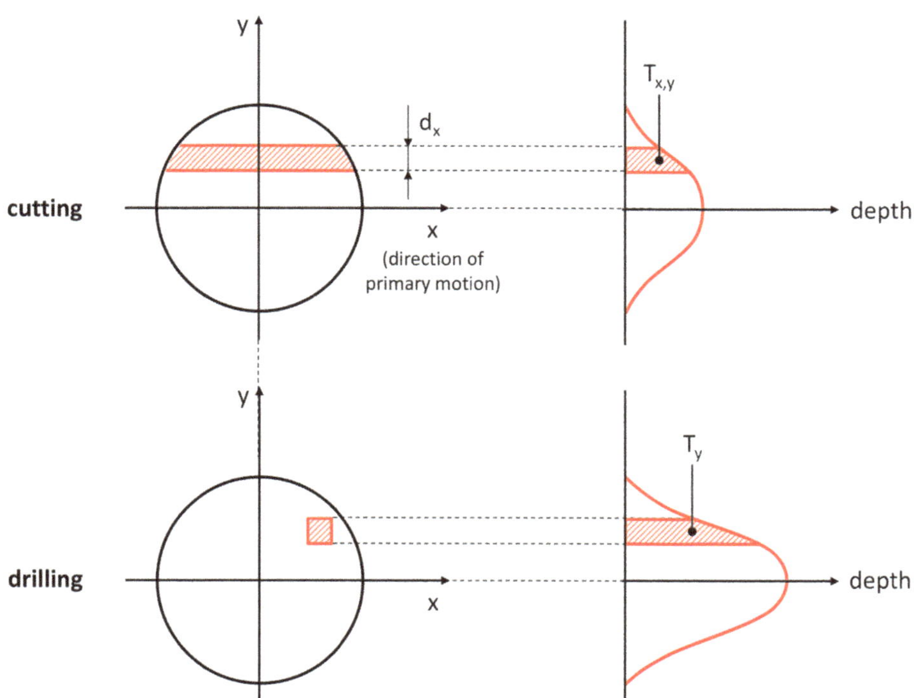

Figure 5.17. Comparison of cutting and drilling depth resulting for laser-induced thermal cutting (top) and drilling (bottom) (adapted from [16]).

As an approach, drilling could be referred to as cutting without any relative speed between the laser outlet nozzle and the 'work piece' tissue. The cutting speed v_{cut} is thus 0. In this case, equation (5.5) can be rewritten as

$$d^{(x,y)} = I^{(x,y)} \cdot t \tag{5.6}$$

as long as the intensity remains constant. The drilling depth then directly represents the intensity profile of the incoming laser beam. When varying the focus diameter $2w_0$ of the laser beam, the intensity (= power per area, where the area follows from the focus diameter) and the drilling depth are altered[21]. This proportionality can be written as

$$d \propto I \propto \frac{1}{2w_0^2}. \tag{5.7}$$

In the case of cutting, the laser beam is moved at a certain velocity, i.e. the above-mentioned cutting speed v_{cut}, over the bone or tissue. The intensity is thus not only dependent on the x- and y-coordinate, i.e. the position on the bone or tissue, but also on time as introduced by the motion of the laser beam over the tissue. When substituting the term dt by $1/v_{\mathrm{cut}}\, dx$, equation (5.5) can be rewritten as

$$d^{(y)} = \frac{1}{v_{\mathrm{cut}}} \int I_{(x)}^{(y)} dx \tag{5.8}$$

as long as the cutting speed v_{cut} is constant and higher than 0. Note that in this example expressed by equation (5.8), the direction of primary motion is given by the x-axis shown in figure 5.17(top). As a result of the integration in x-direction, the cutting depth is

$$d \propto \sqrt{I} \propto \frac{1}{2w_0}. \tag{5.9}$$

It finally turns out that in contrast to the drilling depth, the cutting depth is proportional to the reciprocal value of the focus diameter. This is expressed by a linear relationship, but not a quadratic one as valid in the case of drilling.

The cutting speed can be determined on the basis of the assumption that tissue material is removed if two essential requirements are fulfilled. First, the boiling point or vaporisation temperature T_v has to be reached and second, latent heat of vaporisation L_v has to be delivered continuously once the boiling point has been reached. In this model, secondary effects such as heat dissipation by blood flow or absorption of laser light by the vapour formed above the operating field are neglected. In this case, a phase boundary between the vapour (gaseous phase) and tissue (solid phase) or—eventually—molten material (liquid phase) can be defined. For the idealised case of constant process parameters and static optical properties of

[21] For instance, the intensity is reduced by a factor of four when increasing the focus diameter by a factor of two.

the involved media, this phase boundary propagates into the material to be ablated (here: tissue or bone) with a constant ablation speed v_{abl}, given by

$$v_{abl} = \frac{I}{\rho \cdot [c \cdot (T_v - T_0) + L_v]}. \qquad (5.10)$$

Here, I is the intensity of the incoming laser irradiation, ρ is the density of the irradiated tissue, c is its specific heat capacity and T_0 is the initial temperature, usually body temperature. The relevant constants of water applied for the approximated calculation of the ablation speed of biological tissue are listed in table 5.2.

5.6.2 Cutting of bones

The conventional method for cutting bones is the use of a classic mechanical saw. As a result, merely straight and comparatively wide and non-regular, i.e. chipped and flaked, cuts can be realised. Moreover, the tissue is impacted by the frictional heat which arises during sawing and metallic saw dust and bone debris are produced. This metallic saw dust may distort subsequently taken magnetic resonance images and the bone debris has to be removed from the wound prior to its closure. These disturbing effects can be avoided when cutting bones with the use of lasers where pulsed carbon dioxide lasers are employed most frequently. The application of such laser irradiation at high repetition rate and in the far infrared wavelength range causes an explosion-like vaporisation of bone liquid, whereas the neighbouring tissue is not affected by heat. Employing lasers for cutting bones thus features some advantages such as for example a decrease in adverse effects for the patient and an improved and faster adhesion of the cut bones in comparison to the conventional, mechanical method.

5.6.3 Cutting of tissue

The conventional methods for cutting tissue are the use of scalpels or high-frequency cutting electrodes. In the latter case, the electrical current within the electrode causes extremely fast heating of the tissue. Due to such fast heating, the interstitial fluid is not vaporised moderately, but a high vapour pressure is induced, leading to explosive disruption of the tissue. This process occurs in a locally selective manner, the cuts realised in this way are thus on a microscopic scale. The use of cutting

Table 5.2. Relevant constants of water applied for the calculation of the ablation speed of biological tissue according to equation (5.10).

Parameter	Value
Density ρ	1 kg dm^{-3}
Specific heat capacity c	4.187 kJ kg^{-1} K^{-1}
Vaporisation temperature T_v	100°C
Latent heat for vaporisation L_v	2.26 kJ g^{-1}

electrodes consequently represents an effective and precise method for cutting electrically conductive tissue. However, lasers have replaced this approach in some applications due to the possibility of even more precise and local treatment which is made possible by the use of hot tips or bare fibres, see section 2.3.1.

As presented in detail in section 3.2, the thermal impact of laser irradiation on tissue is based on the absorption[22] and conversion of the incoming optical laser energy into heat energy. Depending on the tissue's absorption, a certain power per volume is absorbed, resulting in the storage of heat energy within the tissue. As a consequence, the tissue is heated where its heat capacity is the dominating parameter which gives the final temperature. According to Beer–Lambert law (see section 3.1.1), the absorbed energy decreases with increasing penetration depth. This therefore also applies for temperature. Moreover, a portion of incoming laser light is scattered and thus causes an increase in temperature of the surrounding tissue volume which is not directly exposed to laser irradiation. At the same time, the irradiated area is cooled via heat dissipation by blood flow as presented in more detail in section 3.1.3. As a result of these interacting phenomena—direct absorption and heating, scattering and indirect heating, and heat dissipation—a temperature gradient is formed within the tissue. In order to initiate laser-induced cutting, a temperature of approximately 300 °C has to be obtained, whereas coagulation already occurs at a temperature of approximately 60 °C[23]. An overview of heat-induced effects on tissue is shown in figure 3.29 and listed in table 5.3.

Table 5.3. Overview of thermal effects and optical and mechanical modifications of tissue induced by an increase in temperature [11].

Temperature in °C	Thermal effect	Optical modification	Mechanical modification
37–60	Heating	None	None
60–65	Thermal denaturation of albumen	Off-white colouring and increase in scattering	Disaggregation
90–100	Drying	Constant maximum scattering	Shrinking and fluid loss
> 150	Carbonisation	Black colouring and increase in absorption	Severe mechanical damage
> 300	Vaporisation and burn	Formation of smoke	Removal

[22] The nature and amount of absorption depends on both the type of tissue and the laser wavelength. In the ultraviolet, visible and near infrared wavelength range absorption is mainly due to interactions of the electromagnetic field of laser light and electrons within the tissue. Conversion into heat subsequently occurs due to collisions and radiationless relaxation. In contrast, the excitation of rotational or vibrational states of molecules is the underlying mechanism for absorption in the infrared wavelength range. The optical energy is then converted into heat energy during the relaxation of excited molecules.

[23] Normally, no irreversible damage occurs up to a tissue temperature of 45 °C.

However, one has to consider that the exposure time, i.e. the duration of laser irradiation and the resulting heat input[24], plays an essential role, as discussed in more detail in section 3.2.2. Moreover, the optical, thermal and mechanical properties of tissue are altered when exposed to laser irradiation, depending on the resulting increase in temperature (see table 5.3). In particular, the time-dependent process of carbonisation and the accompanying blackening significantly impacts the absorption characteristics. This also applies to the drying of tissue since in this case the water content and consequently the absorption characteristics as well as the heat conductivity of tissue are altered, giving rise to heat accumulation. All the effects listed in table 5.3 occur in the course of a laser cutting process of tissue. At the centre of the beam profile of the incoming laser beam which is most frequently Gaussian distributed, tissue is vaporised once a temperature of 300 °C is reached or exceeded. Moreover, the neighbouring tissue layer where the temperature amounts to 150 °C is carbonised. This layer is followed by a further one where the tissue is coagulated. Both layers, the so-called carbonisation edge and the coagulation edge, represent irreversible tissue damage. The thickness of these layers mainly depends on the type of tissue as well as the wavelength and power or energy density and depth of penetration of the incoming laser irradiation, but is also influenced by secondary parameters such as the properties of the surrounding medium and the burn-off, also known as ablation plume, i.e. the laser-ablated and ejected tissue material[25]. An overview on these parameters is given in table 5.4.

For instance, the burn-off products directly impact the width of the carbonisation edge and the coagulation edge during the vaporisation of tissue via carbon dioxide lasers. Both the prevention of a carbonisation edge and the formation of a narrow coagulation edge are achieved when applying a gas jet simultaneously to the actual laser cutting process. This gas jet removes the burn-off products from the cutting zone and thus contributes significantly to the quality of the resulting cut[26].

In addition to the above-mentioned edges, another layer where the tissue is heated and temporarily affected, but not irreversibly damaged, is found at the outer rim of the zone of interaction between the incoming laser beam and the tissue, as shown in figure 5.18.

In the case of cutting with carbon dioxide lasers, the cutting process is based on the strong absorption of water within the tissue for the incident laser irradiation. Here, the depth of penetration is lower than 100 μm. As a consequence, the use of

[24] For instance, a short-term heating of tissue up to a temperature of 70 °C for a duration of just one second causes similar damage as a comparatively long-term heating up to a temperature of 58 °C for a duration of ten seconds.

[25] The ablation plume may have a severe impact on the incoming laser irradiation, e.g. by scattering or shadowing or even focussing or defocussing. This is due to the fact that the ablation plume consists of tissue particles (= absorbers and scatter centres) and free electrons, depending on the laser pulse duration and ablation mechanism. Dense ablation plumes with a high number of electrons are even capable of absorbing incident laser irradiation.

[26] The width of the coagulation edge is approximately 100 μm when introducing a gas jet to carbon dioxide laser cutting of tissue. In contrast, its width is approximately ten times higher (1 mm) for pure cutting without any gas jet.

Table 5.4. Overview of parameters influencing the interaction of laser irradiation with tissue and the accompanying material removal as well as the formation of carbonisation and coagulation edges, respectively.

Category	Parameters
Incoming laser beam	Wavelength
	Power/energy density (following from laser power/energy and beam diameter)
	Operating mode (cw or pulsed)
	Pulse duration (for pulsed operation)
	Pulse shape (for pulsed operation)
	Repetition rate (for pulsed operation)
	etc
Surrounding medium	Index of refraction (and resulting reflectance at interface medium-tissue)
Air	
Water	Transmittance (and accompanying attenuation of laser power/energy)
Blood	
Body liquids	Homogeneity (and resulting loss in laser power/energy due to scattering)
Ablation plume	Temperature (and resulting focussing, or defocussing)
	Transmittance (and accompanying attuation of laser power/energy)
	Electron density (and resulting absorption)
	Stream characteristics (and resulting inhomogeneity in index of refraction)
	etc
Tissue	Index of refraction (and resulting at interface medium-tissue)
	Absorption (and resulting depth of penetration of incident laser irradiation)
	Scattering characteristics
	Heat capacity
	Heat conductivity
	Humidity
	etc

this type of laser allows the cutting and removal of thin slices. The cutting speed strongly depends on the laser intensity since a certain constant energy per unit length[27] has to be maintained in the course of the process for effective cutting. Finally, carbon dioxide lasers feature poor coagulation properties where the maximum size of vessels which can be closed steadily is approximately 500 µm. In contrast to carbon dioxide laser irradiation, a Nd:YAG laser beam penetrates much deeper into the tissue. The resulting effects differ significantly. For instance, tissue

[27] The energy per unit length E is given by the ratio of the laser power P and the cutting speed v_{cut}, $E = P/v_{cut}$.

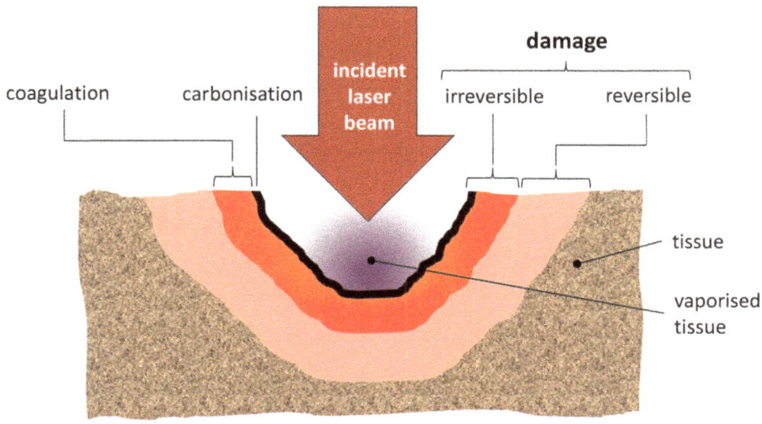

Figure 5.18. Overview of laser-induced impact on tissue including the characteristic resulting zones and edges (adapted from [16]).

cannot be immediately vaporised at moderate laser irradiation (i.e. approximately 30 W) due to low absorption and high scattering, leading to a chaotic diffusion of incident laser light and thus inhibiting its concentration within a small volume. Hence, only the coagulation of tissue occurs at short treatment times. In contrast, Nd:YAG laser irradiation causes a heating and accompanying drying of the tissue if applied for longer treatment times; such drying finally results in a decrease in heat conductivity and a further increase in temperature of the irradiated tissue. This process induces carbonisation which is accompanied by a darkening of the tissue and consequently an increase in its absorbance. Finally, the incoming laser beam is completely absorbed within a thin tissue surface layer which is abruptly vaporised.

However, this process of vaporisation does not take place at low laser power since the laser energy is completely dissipated into the surrounding tissue due to heat conduction and dissipation. In this case, only coagulation is obtained. This fact may appear disadvantageous, but can be used for closing vessels with a diameter of up to 5 mm by laser-induced coagulation and shrinking due to the high depth of penetration of laser irradiation. Effective cutting of tissue is achieved above a laser power of approximately 70 W when working with standard focussing handpieces at low cutting speed. One of the main advantages of the use of Nd:YAG laser irradiation in the near wavelength range is the possibility of laser beam guidance within optical fibres. In combination with different contact tips as presented in section 2.3, this allows the extravascular or intravascular application of laser light either in contacting or non-contacting operation, as shown in figure 5.19.

Non-contacting operation can be realised by fibres which provide divergent beams or with the aid of focussing handpieces. In the latter case, the laser beam's focal diameter and the power/energy density, respectively, can furthermore be adjusted in order to achieve either coagulation or vaporisation. The large coagulation edge resulting in the course of non-contacting vaporisation allows effective haemostasis where veins and arteries with maximum diameters of 3 and 1.5 mm, respectively, can be closed steadily. Much smaller coagulation edges and high

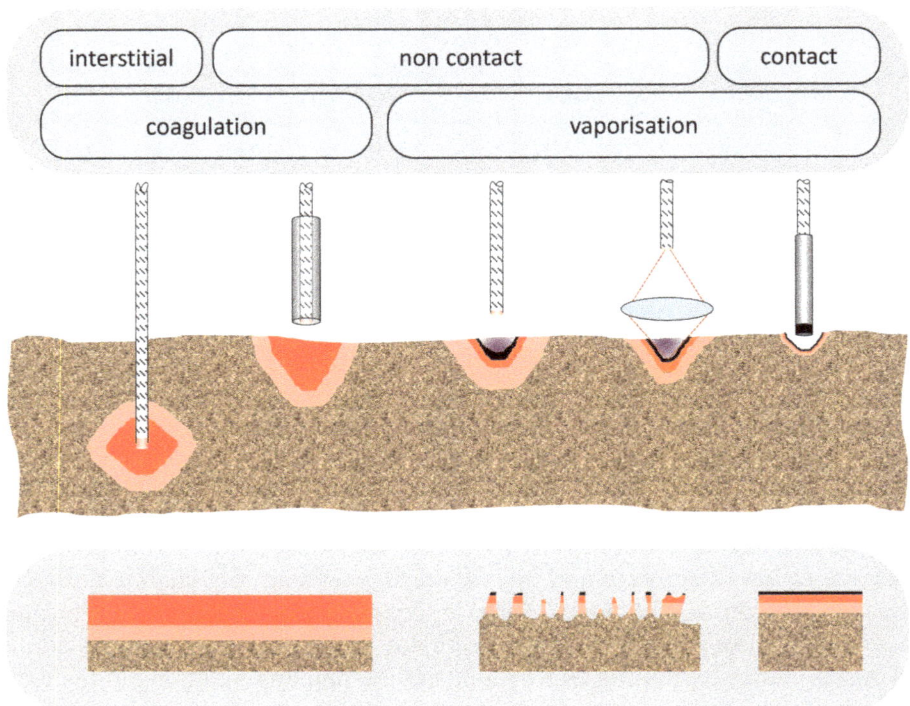

Figure 5.19. Overview of different approaches of Nd:YAG laser treatment of tissue (adapted from [16]).

cutting quality are achieved when applying bare fibres. Here, a carbonised layer is formed at the contact zone between the fibre end face and the tissue, resulting in an increased absorption of incident laser light. When working with Nd:YAG lasers, the penetration depth of photons is thus notably decreased and a similar mode of operation to that found for carbon dioxide lasers is obtained.

5.7 Lasers in dermatology

5.7.1 Treatment of varicose veins

The vein system and venous diseases

In the blood circuit, the veins transport blood with low oxygen content from the tissue to the heart and the lungs where it is enriched again with oxygen and brought back to the tissue via the arteries. At the bottom of the human body, the legs[28] and the feet, the transport from the tissue to the heart has to overcome the force of gravity. This is achieved by venous valves which could be compared to non-return valves, thus inhibiting the reflux of blood towards the legs due to gravity. Opening of

[28] The legs feature a so-called deep vein system and a superficial vein system. The first one collects blood from deeper regions of the muscles and transports 80% of the entire blood volume, whereas the latter transports 20% of the blood volume from the tissue and near-surface regions of the muscles.

these valves in the flow direction follows from the heart's pumping force and the movement of the leg muscles[29]. A malfunction or damage of this venous valve system initially leads to pathological changes of the superficial and the deep vein system, followed by irreversible damage of tissue and musculature.

Venous diseases are frequent health issues in developed western nations[30] where approximately 40% of women and 20% of men suffer from symptoms induced by such diseases. In severe cases, even open and non-healing wounds or phlebitis and vein thrombosis can occur. However, typical symptoms are less dangerous and include feelings of heaviness as well as pain and swelling of the legs. But also cosmetic aspects such as permanent discolouration, leading to unattractive legs and an eventually accompanying psychological stress have to be considered. This also applies for the widespread varicose veins. In most cases (95%), such varicose veins are due to a congenital weakness of the vein walls and the connective tissue. If too much blood remains within the legs, e.g. in the case of longer motionlessness during sitting, the veins are expanded until the venous valve cannot close the expanded veins. The valve can thus not meet its function, resulting in a flow reversal of blood towards the legs and feet due to gravity. This effect is also referred to as blow-out and can take place for years without being noticed. In the course of time, the blow-out increases since the number of expanded veins and dysfunctional venous valves increases. This creeping process finally leads to the formation of varicose veins, either by accumulation of blood within superficial veins (i.e. the actual or primary varicose vein) or by a blocking of the blood flow within the deeper vein system, e.g. by a thrombus or a tumour, and the subsequent formation of a bypass blood circuit via superficial veins. This leads to a further expansion of these veins and causes the so-called secondary varicose vein.

Varicose veins are not only defective in appearance, but also represent a considerable disease which may cause severe damage in the affected leg due to an inhibited blood flow, mainly occurring in the distal lower leg. Initially, non-specific symptoms as mentioned above, heaviness and swelling of the legs, as well as cramps in the calf and pruritus are noticed. At the more advanced stage, cicatrisation of skin, subcutaneous tissue, and fascia can occur. Other possible and severe consequences are thrombophlebitis or even ulcus cruris venosum.

The classical approach for the removal of varicose veins is vein stripping [25, 26]. Here, affected veins are extricated from the leg using a probe. This method is suitable for removing main, truncal varicose veins and for treating smaller branches and spider veins, also known as idiopathic telangiectases, by injection. Moreover, the technique of radiofrequency treatment is in hand where the affected vein is treated by heat supplied by a thermo element which is brought into the vein via a catheter. Another comparatively novel approach is the endovenous laser treatment

[29] For instance, the rhythmic movement during walking or jogging leads to a periodical extension and contraction of leg muscles, the leg musculature thus acts as a pump.

[30] Here, the professional life is frequently dominated by seated activities, leading to prolonged sitting (or standing in some cases).

(ELT) or endovenous/endoluminal laser therapy [27] as described in the following section.

Endovenous/endoluminal laser therapy

In the course of minimal-invasive endovenous/endoluminal laser therapy, varicose veins are treated by incident laser light where the light energy is converted into heat energy due to absorption at haemoglobin [28]. This leads to an increase in temperature within the treated vein, e.g. the great saphenous vein, up to approximately 60–70 °C and an accompanying modification and shrinking of the inner vein wall as well as a blood clotting within the vein. The vein's cross section is consequently reduced and the modified tissue is subsequently dissolved by the body's own decomposition enzymes. For this technique, pulsed or continuous wave diode lasers with an emission wavelength of 810 nm, 940 nm and 980 nm are used [29–32]. The transport of laser light is achieved by puncturing the affected vein and inserting an optical fibre. The actual operating field is previously identified and located via ultrasonic monitoring, which is additionally applied for accurate positioning of the fibre end in the course of the surgical intervention. Moreover, the affected region of the vein is locally anaesthetised.

In comparison to classical vein stripping, endovenous/endoluminal laser therapy stands out due to a number of advantages such as a marginal degree of intervention (by punctuation), a reduced risk of postoperative bleeding or infection of the wound, and improved cosmetic results. However, this laser-based method might not be sufficient in severe cases where additional removal of affected branches via mini-phlebectomy is required.

5.7.2 Removal of tattoos

In recent years, tattoos have become socially acceptable and the number of tattoos has increased significantly. Although a tattoo is quite easy to realise, its removal is much more difficult. However, the techniques used here have been improved notably in the last decade. Particularly painful methods[31] which were accompanied with scarring were replaced by modern laser processes. This was made possible by the further development of pulsed laser sources. The wide range of available wavelengths allows the removing of tattoos on the basis of selective photo-thermolysis, i.e. the localised thermal destruction of specific chromophores within the skin. This selectivity is due to the fact that such chromophores, for example melanin or haemoglobin, feature notably different absorption characteristics. The particular laser used and its wavelength has to be selected on the basis of the absorption maximum of the chromophore to be removed, brightened or bleached. Further, the laser source should be pulsed and the pulse duration should be shorter than the thermal relaxation time of the chromophore of interest. An overview on laser

[31] As an example, dermabrasion can be used for the removal of tattoos. However, this method cannot be applied in the case of thin skin. Another method is vaporisation of the skin by carbon dioxide laser irradiation.

Table 5.5. Selection of pulsed laser sources frequently used for the removal of tattoos [33–36].

Laser type	Wavelength in nm	Pulse duration in ns
2nd Harmonic Nd:YAG laser	532	5–7
Ruby laser(Q-switched)	694	25–40
Alexandrite laser(Q-switched)	755	50–100
Nd:YAG laser(Q-switched)	1064	5–7

Table 5.6. Grades of brightening used for evaluating the success of laser-induced removal of tattoos.

Grade of brightening	Share of removed tattoo ink pigments in %
Complete brightening	100
Very good brightening	70–99
Good brightening	40–69
Poor brightening	< 40

sources frequently used for selective photo-thermolysis and the accompanying removal of tattoos is given in table 5.5.

For instance, both the ruby laser and the 2nd harmonic Nd:YAG laser have turned out to be suitable for the removal of black tattoos since such laser light is extremely well absorbed by black and green ink pigments [37]. However, this also bears the risk of inducing pigmentary abnormality due to the fact that red and green laser light is also well absorbed by the body's own melanin. This effect can be avoided when working with near infrared laser irradiation such as for example the fundamental wavelength of Q-switched Nd:YAG lasers of 1064 nm. Laser irradiation at this wavelength exhibits a high penetration depth into tissue and a negligible interaction with melanin-containing cells [33]. In contrast, it is well absorbed by the pigments of black ink. Black, deep purple and green pigments can also be efficiently removed by alexandrite lasers [35].

For the laser-induced removal of tattoos, the skin is usually anaesthetised locally by applying an anaesthetic cream such as for example a mixture of lidocaine and prilocaine about one to three hours prior to the actual laser application. In case of bleeding or vesication within the irradiated skin, the irradiated area is dressed with sulfadiazine-containing bandages. In order to evaluate the success of a laser treatment, the grade of brightening is taken as a basis, as listed in table 5.6.

5.8 Lasers in therapy—the bottom line

- Reduced swelling power of intervertebral discs may lead to the rupture of the fibrocartilage and the leakage of the gelatinous disc core.
- Percutaneous laser disk decompression (PLDD) is a micro-surgical method for the treatment of disc lesions.

- Kidney stones result from the crystallisation of substances from the urine as a consequence of dehydration, poor or wrong nutrition, immobilisation, or urinary tract infections.
- Kidney and gall stones can be fragmented and removed by laser-induced shock wave lithotripsy (LISL) where cracking of stones is due to the mechanical force provided by laser-induced shock waves.
- The human eye is a complex imaging system and basically consists of the eye ball, the eye lens for focussing of incident light, and the retina for light detection.
- Per definition, the standardised distance of most distinct vision amounts to 25 cm.
- The eye's optical power is given in dioptres.
- Laser assisted *in situ* keratomileusis (LASIK) is a method for the reduction of defective vision via re-shaping the cornea by laser irradiation.
- The minimal-invasive method of laser-induced thermotherapy (LITT) is applied for the treatment of malignant and benignant tumours by inducing interstitial coagulation.
- The efficiency of laser-induced thermotherapy is increased by using the so-called power mode where treatment starts at high laser power which is subsequently stepwise reduced.
- Excimer laser-assisted non-occlusive anastomosis (ELANA) is an alternative method for bypass operation for the abatement of symptoms caused by aneurysms. It allows bypass surgery without interrupting the blood supply of the brain.
- Transmyocardial laser revascularisation (TMLR) is a laser-based therapy method applied for improving in the perfusion of the heart by drilling a number of channels into the myocardial muscle.
- Lasers are suitable for cutting and drilling bones and tissue and even allow the reduction of disturbing effects such as, for example, the formation of saw dust or extreme bleeding which may occur in the case of classical methods.
- The application of laser irradiation not only allows cutting and drilling via vaporisation, but also drying and coagulation of tissue and the removal of thin tissue layers.
- During laser cutting of tissue, the exposure time and the resulting heat input play an essential role where the optical and thermal properties of the particular tissue and the surrounding medium have to be considered additionally.
- In dermatology, the method of minimal-invasive endovenous/endoluminal laser therapy allows the treatment of varicose veins by laser-induced shrinking of the inner walls of affected veins.
- Lasers are suitable for the removal of tattoos by selective photo-thermolysis where the tattoo ink pigments are decomposed or bleached as evaluated on the basis of the resulting grade of brightening.

References

[1] Schenk B, Brouwer P, Peul W and van Buchem M 2006 *Am. J. Neuroradiol.* **27** 232–5

[2] Ascher P W, Choy D S and Yuri H 1989 *Lasers Surg. Med. Suppl.* **1** 48–8

[3] Choy D S J 2001 *J. Clin. Laser Med. Surg.* **19** 231–3

[4] Gevargez A, Groenemeyer D W and Czerwinski F 2000 *Eur. Radiol.* **10** 1239–41

[5] Wondrazek F and Frank F 1988 Devices for intracorporal laser-induced shock-wave lithotripsy (ilisl) *Laser Lithotripsy* ed R W Steiner (Berlin, Heidelberg: Springer), 123–8 pp ISBN 978-3-642-73864-7

[6] Rink K, Delacrïétaz G and Salathïé R P 1995 *Lasers Surg Med.* 134–46

[7] Fuh E, Haleblian G E, Norris R D, Albala W D M, Simmons N, Zhong P and Preminger G M 2007 *J. Urol.* **177** 1542–5

[8] Hochberger J, Tex S, Bayer J, Stein R, Tschepe J and Hahn E G 1997 *Biomed. Tech.* **42** 331–31

[9] Zörcher T, Hochberger J, Schrott K-M, Kühn R and Schafhauser W 1999 *Lasers Surg. Med.* **25** 38–42

[10] Chang A W, Tsang A C, Contreras J E, Huynh P D, Calvano C J, Crnic-Rein T C and Thall E H 2003 *J. Cataract Refract. Surg.* **29** 1204–10

[11] Berlien H P and Muller G 2000 *Angewandte Lasermedizin—Lehr und Handbuch für Praxis und Klinik* 3rd edn (Berlin: Laser- und Medizin-Technologie) ISBN 3-609-70510-8

[12] Sekundo W, Kunert K S and Blum M 2011 *Br. J. Ophthalmol.* **95** 335–9

[13] Blum M, Kunert K, Schröder M and Sekundo W 2010 *Graefeas Arch. Clin. Exp. Ophthalmol.* **248** 1019–27

[14] Li M, Zhou Z, Shen Y, Knorz M C, Gong L and Zhou X 2014 *J. Refrac. Surg.* **30** 94–100

[15] Kertes P J and Johnson T M 2007 *Evidence-based Eye Care* (Philadelphia, PA: Lippincott Williams & Wilkins)

[16] Berlien H P and Muller G 2003 *Applied Laser Medicine* (Berlin Heidelberg: Springer Verlag) ISBN 978-3-642-62391-2

[17] Müller G J and Roggan A 1995 *Laser Induced Interstitial Thermotherapy* (Bellingham, WA: SPIE, The International Society for Optical Engineering)

[18] Langer D J and Vajkoczy P 2005 *Skull Base* **15** 191–205

[19] Langer D J, Zwan A V D, Vajkoczy P, Kivipelto L, Doormaal T P V and Tulleken C A F 2008 *Neurosurgical Focus* **24** E6

[20] van Doormaal T P C, van der Zwan A, Verweij B H, Regli L and Tulleken C A F 2010 *Neurosurgery* **66** 439–47

[21] van Doormaal T P, van der Zwan A, Verweij B H, Han K S, Langer D J and Tulleken C A 2008 *Neurosurgery* **63** 12–22

[22] Lutter G, Saurbier B, Nitzsche E, Kletzin F, Martin J, Schlensak C, Lutz C and Beyersdorf F 1998 *Eur. J. Cardiothorac Surg.* **13** 21–26

[23] Lange R A and Hillis L D 1999 *New Engl. J. Med.* **341** 1075–6

[24] Horvath K A 2004 *Curr. Treat. Opt. Cardiovasc. Med.* **6** 53–9

[25] Dwerryhouse S, Davies B, Harradine K and Earnshaw J J 1999 *J. Vasc. Surg.* **29** 589–92

[26] Rasmussen L, Lawaetz M, Bjoern L, Vennits B, Blemings A and Eklof B 2011 *Br. J. Surg.* **98** 1079–87

[27] Sroka R, Weick K, Sadeghi-Azandaryani M, Steckmeier B and Schmedt C G 2010 *J. Biophoton.* **3** 269–76

[28] Navarro L, Min R J and Boné C 2001 *Dermatol. Surg.* **27** 117–22

[29] Min R J, Khilnani N and Zimmet S E 2003 *J. Vasc. Interv. Radiol.* **14** 991–6
[30] Proebstle T M, Krummenauer F, Gül D and Knop J 2004 *Dermatol. Surg.* **30** 174–8
[31] Agus G, Mancini S and Magi G 2006 *Int. Angiol.* **25** 209–15
[32] Proebstle T, Lehr H, Kargl A, Espinola-Klein C, Rother W, Bethge S and Knop J 2002 *J. Vasc. Surg.* **35** 729–36
[33] Tammaro A, Fatuzzo G, Narcisi A, Abruzzese C, Caperchi C, Gamba A, Parisella F and Persechino S 2012 *Int. J. Immunopathol. Pharmacol.* **25** 537–9
[34] Kilmer S L and Anderson R 1993 *J. Dermatol. Surgery Oncol.* **19** 330–8
[35] Alster T S 1995 *J. Am. Acad. Dermatol.* **33** 69–73
[36] Scheibner A, Kenny G, White W and Wheeland R G 1990 *J. Dermatol. Surgery Oncol.* **16** 1091–8
[37] Kilmer S L, Lee M S, Grevelink J M, Flotte T J and Anderson R R 1993 *Arch. Dermatol.* **129** 971–8

IOP Publishing

Lasers in Medical Diagnosis and Therapy
Basics, applications and future prospects
Stephan Wieneke and Christoph Gerhard

Appendix A

A.1 Formulary

Chapter 1—Laser basics

Photon energy of a light wave

$$E_{\text{Photon}} = h \cdot f$$

h: Planck's constant ($h = 6.626 \cdot 10^{-34}$ m^2 kg s^{-1}),
f: frequency [s^{-1}].

Wavelength

$$\lambda = \frac{c_0}{f} = \frac{c_0 \cdot h}{E_2 - E_1}$$

c_0: The speed of light in vacuum ($c_0 = 3 \times 10^8$ m s^{-1}),
E_2, E_1: Energy level [J].

Resonator condition

$$\lambda = \frac{2 \cdot l_r}{N}$$

l_r: length of laser resonator [m],
N: integer.

Chapter 2—Basics of medical laser systems

Distribution of refractive index over radius of a GRIN lens

$$n(r) = n_{\text{centre}} \cdot \sec(g \cdot r)$$

doi:10.1088/978-0-7503-1275-2ch6

n_{centre}: index of refraction at lens centre,
sec: hyperbolic secant distribution,
g: geometrical gradient constant,
r: radius.

Critical angle of total internal reflection

$$\alpha_{\text{tot}} = \arcsin \frac{n_2}{n_1}$$

n_2: index of refraction of optically thin medium,
n_1: index of refraction of optically dense medium.

Critical entrance angle of light

$$\alpha_{\max} = \arcsin\left(\sqrt{n_{\text{core}}^2 - n_{\text{cladding}}^2}\right)$$

n_{core}: index of refraction of fibre core,
n_{cladding}: index of refraction of fibre cladding.

Numerical aperture

$$\text{NA} = n_{\text{a}} \cdot \sin \alpha_{\max}$$

n_{a}: index of refraction of ambient medium.

Fibre damping

$$D = 10 \cdot \frac{1}{l} \log \frac{P_{\text{in}}}{P(l)}$$

l: length (of light path within optical fibre),
P_{in}: initial power of incident light,
$P(l)$: power of light at position l.

Number of modes guided within a bent fibre

$$N_g = N_0 \cdot \left(1 - \frac{D_{\text{core}} \cdot n_{\text{cladding}}^2}{R \cdot \text{NA}_0^2}\right)$$

N_0: number of modes guided in fibre without bending
D_{core}: fibre core diameter,
R: bending radius,
NA_0: numerical aperture of fibre without bending.

Effective numerical aperture

$$\mathrm{NA}_{\mathrm{eff}} = \sqrt{n_{\mathrm{core}}^2 - n_{\mathrm{cladding}}^2 \cdot \left(1 + \frac{D_{\mathrm{core}}}{2 \cdot R}\right)^2}$$

Chapter 3—Tissue optics and laser–tissue interactions

Total reflectance

$$R = \frac{I_{\mathrm{R}} + I_{\mathrm{RS}}}{I_0}$$

I_0: initial intensity of incident light,
I_{R}: specular fraction of reflected light,
I_{RS}: diffuse fraction of reflected light.

Total transmittance

$$T = \frac{I_{\mathrm{T}} + I_{\mathrm{TS}}}{I_0}$$

Total absorbance

$$A = \frac{I_0 - I_{\mathrm{R}} - I_{\mathrm{RS}} - I_{\mathrm{T}} - I_{\mathrm{TS}}}{I_0}$$

Snell's law (of refraction)

$$\sin\alpha_1 \cdot n_1 = \sin\alpha_2 \cdot n_2$$

α_1: angle of incidence,
n_1: index of refraction in front of interface,
α_2: refraction angle,
n_2: index of refraction behind interface.

Reflectance of s-polarised light (Fresnel equation)

$$R_{\mathrm{s-pol}} = \left| \frac{n_1 \cdot \cos\alpha_1 - n_2 \cdot \cos\alpha_2}{n_1 \cdot \cos\alpha_1 + n_2 \cdot \cos\alpha_2} \right|^2$$

Reflectance of p-polarised light (Fresnel equation)

$$R_{\mathrm{p-pol}} = \left| \frac{n_2 \cdot \cos\alpha_1 - n_1 \cdot \cos\alpha_2}{n_2 \cdot \cos\alpha_1 + n_1 \cdot \cos\alpha_2} \right|^2$$

Total reflectance (considering polarisation effects)

$$R_{\text{tot}} = \frac{R_{\text{s-pol}} + R_{\text{p-pol}}}{2}$$

Total reflectance (special case of normal incidence)

$$R_{\text{tot}} = \left(\frac{n_2 - n_1}{n_2 + n_1}\right)^2$$

Transmittance of s-polarised light (Fresnel equation)

$$T_{\text{s-pol}} = \left|\frac{2 \cdot n_1 \cdot \cos\alpha_1}{n_1 \cdot \cos\alpha_1 + n_2 \cdot \cos\alpha_2}\right|^2$$

Transmittance of p-polarised light (Fresnel equation)

$$T_{\text{p-pol}} = \left|\frac{2 \cdot n_1 \cdot \cos\alpha_1}{n_2 \cdot \cos\alpha_1 + n_1 \cdot \cos\alpha_2}\right|^2$$

Beer–Lambert law

$$I_{\text{T}} = I_0 e^{-c_{\text{a}} \cdot \sigma_{\text{a}} \cdot d} = I_0 e^{-\mu_{\text{a}} \cdot d}$$

I_{T}: intensity of transmitted light,
I_0: initial intensity of incident light,
c_{a}: absorber concentration,
σ_{a}: absorption cross section,
μ_{a}: absorption coefficient,
d: thickness of irradiated medium.

Transmitted intensity

$$I_{\text{T}} = I_0 \cdot 10^{-\varepsilon \cdot c \cdot d} = I_0 \cdot 10^{-A}$$

ε: decade molar extinction coefficient,
c: absorption concentration,
A: absorbance.

Optical penetration depth

$$x_{\text{opt}} = \frac{1}{\mu_{\text{a}}}$$

μ_{a}: absorption coefficient.

Albedo

$$a = \frac{\mu_s}{(\mu_s + \mu_a)}$$

μ_s: scattering coefficient.

Effective attenuation coefficient

$$\mu_{eff} = \sqrt{3\mu_a(\mu_a + \acute{\mu}_s)}$$

$\acute{\mu}_s$: effective scattering coefficient.

Effective optical penetration depth

$$x^*_{opt} = \frac{1}{\mu_{eff}}$$

Effective free length of path

$$l_{eff} = \frac{1}{\mu_a + \acute{\mu}_s}$$

Speed of light within a medium

$$c = \frac{c_0}{n}$$

n: refractive index of the medium.

Increase in temperature

$$\Delta T = \frac{Q}{\rho c}$$

Q: absorbed thermal energy per volume unit [J m^{-3}],
ρ: density [kg m^{-3}],
c: specific heat capacity [J kg^{-1} K^{-1}].

Energy density required for heating material to boiling point

$$Q_b = \rho c \Delta T$$

Energy density required for vaporisation

$$Q_v = \rho L_v$$

L_v: latent heat for vaporisation.

Volume vaporised by laser irradiation

$$V = \frac{P}{Q_v + Q_b}$$

P: laser power.

Cutting depth

$$d_{cut} = \frac{P}{2w_0 \cdot v(Q_v + Q_b)}$$

$2w_0$: focus diameter of laser beam,
v: feed speed.

Heat flow

$$\frac{\Delta Q}{\Delta t} = \lambda \cdot A \frac{T_1 - T_2}{l}$$

λ: thermal or heat conductivity [W m^{-1} K^{-1}],
A: area [m^2],
T: temperature [K],
l: length [m].

Perfusion time of blood

$$t_b = \frac{1}{v_b \cdot \rho}$$

v_b: blood circulation rate,
ρ: density of irradiated tissue.

Thermal depth of penetration

$$d_{th} = \sqrt{\kappa t_b}$$

κ: thermal diffusivity.

Depth of thermal diffusion

$$x_{diff} = \sqrt{2 \cdot \frac{\lambda}{\rho \cdot c} \cdot t}$$

t: time.

Thermal diffusion time

$$t_{\text{diff}} = \frac{x_{\text{opt}}^2}{\kappa}$$

Expansion time of thermo-elastic stress wave

$$t_{\text{stress}} = \frac{1}{c_a \mu_a}$$

Ablation depth

$$x_{\text{abl}} = \frac{1}{\mu_a} \ln\left(\frac{\Phi_0}{\Phi_{\text{thr}}}\right)$$

Φ_{thr}: threshold fluence [J cm^{-2}],
Φ_0: applied fluence [J cm^{-2}].

Chapter 4—Lasers in medical diagnosis

Number of incident photons

$$n_a = N_i n_L \sigma_{ik} \Delta x$$

N_i: density of absorbing molecules or atoms,
n_L: total number of incident photons,
σ_{ik}: absorption cross section of transition from energy level E_i to energy level E_k,
$\Delta\ x$: distance covered by incident laser irradiation.

Number of photons emitted due to fluorescence

$$n_{\text{FL}} = N_K A_k$$

N_i, N_k: number of excited molecules or atoms,
A_k: Einstein coefficient for energy state k.

Wavenumber

$$\bar{\nu} = \frac{1}{\lambda}$$

Laser focus diameter

$$2w_0 \cong 2\lambda \frac{f}{D}$$

f: focal length of used optical system,
D: diameter of used optical system (so-called aperture).

f-Number of an optical system

$$f\# = \frac{f}{D}$$

Minimum detectable diameter (optical resolution limit)

$$d = \frac{\lambda}{2 \cdot n \cdot \sin \alpha}$$

Peripheral oxygen saturation (of blood)

$$S_p O_2 = \frac{HbO_2}{HbO_2 + Hb}$$

HbO_2: concentration of oxygenated haemoglobin,
Hb: concentration of deoxygenated haemoglobin.

Chapter 5—Lasers in medical therapy

Dioptric value (ametropia)

$$p = \frac{1}{f}$$

f: focal length of eye lens [m].

Munnerlyn equation

$$t = z^2 \cdot \frac{p}{3}$$

t: thickness of the cornea material to be removed [μm],
z: diameter of material removal zone [mm],
p: dioptric value to be corrected [dpt].

Laser fluence (at position x)

$$F = F_0 \cdot e^{-x/x_{opt}}$$

F_0: initial maximum fluence,
x: position,
x_{opt}: depth of penetration of laser light.

Ablation depth (expressed on basis of fluence)

$$x_{abl} = x_{opt} \cdot \ln \frac{F_{th}}{F_0}$$

Cutting or drilling depth at position (*x*, *y*) of a laser beam profile

$$d^{(x,\,y)} = \int I_t^{(x,\,y)} dt$$

Cutting depth

$$d \propto \sqrt{I} \propto \frac{1}{2w_0}$$

A.2 Exercises

(1) Determine the increase in temperature ΔT of tissue which is exposed to laser irradiation with a pulse peak power of $P_{max} = 50$ W and a pulse duration of $\tau_p = 12$ μs. The tissue features a specific heat capacity of $c = 2.88$ kJ Kg^{-1} K^{-1}, a density of $\rho = 1300$ kg m^{-3}, and an absorption coefficient of $\mu_a = 100$ cm^{-1}. The shape of the irradiated volume can be approximated by a cylinder with a height h which corresponds to the optical penetration depth x_{opt} of the incident laser irradiation and a diameter d which is given by the laser beam diameter $2w_0 = 150$ μm.

Result: 90.68 °C. (Note: The absorbed thermal energy per volume applies to $Q = P_{max} \cdot \tau_p/V$.)

(2) The defective vision of a patient amounts to +8 dpt and should be corrected using classical LASIK. The thickness of the patient's cornea is 479 μm and the pupil diameter is 6.4 mm. The flap which is initially cut and finally placed on the laser-shaped area of the cornea in the course of LASIK should feature a thickness of 160 μm. In order to ensure the stability of the cornea, the cornea thickness underneath the laser-shaped area must amount to 250 μm. Which dioptric value, can be realised for the given values?

Result: $p = 3$ dpt. (Note: The maximum possible removal cornea thickness t results to $t = 479 - 160 - 250$ μ m = 69 μm.)

(3) Determine the thermal depth of penetration of cerebral tissue ($\rho = 1.02$ g ml^{-1}, $\kappa = 1.2 \times 10^{-7} m^2\, s^{-1}$) with a blood circulation rate of $v_b = 0.55$ ml min^{-1} g^{-1}.

Result: $d_{th} = 3.59$ mm. (Note: The perfusion time is about 107 s.)

(4) Real wave guides such as fibres feature certain losses of light due to different damping mechanisms. Such losses within a fibre should be determined for laser irradiation at a wavelength of $\lambda = 702$ nm and a power of $P = 42$ W. The fibre length is 8 m and its damping amounts to $D = 0.2$ dB m^{-1}. Calculate the fraction of transmitted laser power with respect to the initial power (given in %).

Result: fraction $P(l)/P_0 = 85\%$.

(5) A laser is focussed onto tissue; the focus diameter is $2w_0 = 500$ μm (Gaussian profile), the pulse peak power is $P = 2$ W, and the pulse duration amounts to $\tau_p = 100$ ms. Determine the resulting effect of interaction between laser irradiation and tissue (see figure 3.27).

Result: vaporisation ($I \approx 1000$ W cm^{-2}).

(6) Calculate the photon energy (given in joules and electron volts) of excimer laser irradiation at a wavelength of $\lambda = 308$ nm.

Result: $E_{photon} = 6.42 \times 10^{-19}$ J, $E_{eV} = 4$ eV. (Note: 1 eV = 1.602×10^{-19} J.)

(7) Determine the critical angle of total internal reflection of a step index fibre where the indices of refraction are $n_{core} = 1.32$ for the fibre core and $n_{cladding} = 1.307$ for the fibre cladding.

Result: $\alpha_{tot} = 81.95^\circ$.

(8) Determine the critical entrance angle of a fibre where the indices of refraction are $n_{core} = 1.43$ for the fibre core and $n_{cladding} = 1.39$ for the fibre cladding.

Result: $\alpha_{max} = 19.6$.

(9) The diameter of the fibre core of a step index fibre is $D_{core} = 320$ μm; its indices of refraction for the core and cladding are $n_{core} = 1.32$ and $n_{cladding} = 1.307$, respectively. Determine the numerical aperture, NA, of this fibre in case of fibre bending by a radius of $R = 40$ mm.

Result: $NA_{eff} = 0.184$.

(10) An ideal carbon dioxide laser with a Gaussian beam profile and a power of $P = 120$ W is focussed to a diameter of $2w_0 = 800$ μm. Determine the intensity I of laser light within the focus.

Result: $I = 238.7 \times 10^6$ W m^{-2}.

(11) Determine the refraction angle at an interface from air to tissue where the angle of incidence is $\alpha_1 = 38^\circ$. The indices of refraction are $n_{air} = 1$ for air and $n_{tissue} = 1.38$ for tissue.

Result: $\alpha = 26.5^\circ$.

(12) Determine the reflectance R of tissue with an index of refraction of $n_{tissue} = 1.37$ where the surrounding medium is air with $n_{air} = 1$. The angle of incidence is 0° (i.e. normal incidence). The incident light is laser light with a wavelength of $\lambda = 1064$ nm.

Result: $R_{tot} = 0.024 = 2.4\%$.

(13) A tissue sample (ideal absorption) with a thickness of 3 mm and an absorption coefficient of 12 cm^{-1} is irradiated with laser light at an initial intensity of 100 W cm^{-2}. Determine the intensity of the transmitted light.

Result: $I_T = 2.73$ W cm^{-2}.

(14) Determine the optical depth of penetration of tissue with an absorption coefficient of $\mu_a = 200\ cm^{-1}$.

Result: $x_{opt} = 50$ μm.

(15) Calculate the albedo a of tissue with a scattering–absorption ratio of 70/30.

Result: $a = 0.7$.

(16) Calculate the pulse power of a laser with an average power of 1 mW, a pulse repetition rate of 20 MHz, and a pulse duration of 200 ps.

Result: $P_{max} = 0.25$ W. (Note: $E_{pulse} = P_{avg}/f_{rep}$ and $P_{max} = E_{pulse}/\tau_p$.)

(17) Tissue is cut using carbon dioxide laser irradiation at a power of $P = 140$ W. The laser beam focus diameter is $2w_0 = 230$ μm and the feed speed amounts to $v =$ 4 cm s^{-1}. Estimate the resulting cutting depth on the basis of relevant constants of water as given in 5.2.

Result: $d_{cut} \approx 6.6$ mm.

(18) Determine the perfusion time of kidney tissue with a density of $\rho = 1200$ kg m^{-3} and a blood circulation rate of $v_b = 3.4$ ml min^{-1} g^{-1}.

Result: $t_b \approx 15$ ms.

(19) Determine the thermal diffusion length x_{diff} of adipose tissue ($\lambda = 0.3$ W m^{-1} K^{-1}, $c = 1.93$ kJ Kg^{-1} K^{-1}, $\rho = 900$ kg m^{-3}) which is irradiated with a single laser pulse with a duration of 200 ms.

Result: $x_{diff} \approx 260$ μm.

(20) Taking the blow-off model as a basis, which ablation depth results for the ablation of bone with an absorption coefficient of $\mu_a = 1111\ cm^{-1}$ and a threshold fluence of $F_{thr} = 444$ J cm^{-2} where the incident laser irradiation features a fluence of $F_0 = 1200$ J cm^{-2}?

Result: $x_{abl} \approx 9$ μm.

(21) Determine the focus diameter of a laser scanning microscope where the wavelength of the used light is $\lambda = 532$ nm ($f\# = 3.2$).

Result: $d = 3.4$ μm.

(22) Determine the oxygen saturation within blood where a HbO_2 concentration of 9.2 mmol l^{-1} and a Hb concentration of 0.188 mmol l^{-1} was measured via pulse oximetry.

Result: $S_pO_2 = 0.98$.

A.3 Further reading

Books

Berlien H-P, Müller G J, Breuer H, Krasner N and Okunata T (ed) 2012 *Applied Laser Medicine* (Berlin Heidelberg: Springer)
Dixon J A 1987 *Surgical Application of Lasers* (Maryland Heights, MO: Mosby Publishing)
Eichler J and Seiler T 1993 *Lasertechnik in der Medizin* (Berlin Heidelberg: Springer) (in German)
Goldberg D (ed) 2013 *Laser Dermatology* (Berlin Heidelberg: Springer)
Jelinkova H 2013 *Lasers for Medical Applications* (Swaston: Woodhead Publishing Ltd)
Niemz M H 2007 *Laser–Tissue Interactions: Fundamentals and Applications* (Berlin Heidelberg: Springer)
Nouri K 2012 *Lasers in Dermatology and Medicine* (Berlin Heidelberg: Springer)
Raulin C and Karsai S (ed) 2011 *Laser and IPL Technology in Dermatology and Aesthetic Medicine* (Berlin Heidelberg: Springer)
Wax A and Backman V 2009 *Biomedical Applications of Light Scattering* (New York: McGraw-Hill)
Waynan R W (ed) 2002 *Lasers in Medicine* (Boca Raton, FL: CRC Press)
Weingeist T A 1992 *Laser Surgery in Ophthalmology: Practical Applications* (New York: Appleton and Lange)
Wolbarsht M L (ed) 1971 *Laser Applications in Medicine and Biology* (Berlin Heidelberg: Springer)

Journals

American Journal of Ophthalmology (Elsevier).
Lasers in Medical Science (Springer).
Lasers in Surgery and Medicine (Wiley).
Ophthalmic Surgery, Lasers and Imaging Retina (Wyanoke Group).
Photomedicine and Laser Surgery (Mary Ann Liebert, Inc. publishers).
The Journal of Japan Society for Laser Surgery and Medicine (Japan Society for Laser Surgery and Medicine, JSLSM).

Recommended review articles (selection)

Alam M, Hsu T-S, Dover J S, Wrone D A and Arndt K A 2003 Nonablative laser and light treatments: histology and tissue effects—a review *Lasers Surg. Med.* **33** 30–9

Balles M W, Puliafito C A, D'Amico D J, Jacobsen J J and Birngruber R 1990 Semiconductor diode laser photocoagulation in retinal vascular diseas *Ophthalmology* **97** 1553–61

Basford J R 1995 Low intensity laser therapy: still not an established clinical tool *Lasers Surg. Med.* **16** 331–42

Bass L S and Treat M R 1995 Laser tissue welding: a comprehensive review of current and future *Lasers Surg. Med.* **17** 315–49

Bjordal J M, Coupp C, Chow R T, Tunr J and Ljunggren E A 2003 A systematic review of low level laser therapy with location-specific doses for pain from chronic joint disorders *J. Physiother.* **49** 107–16

Bjordal J M, Johnson M I, Iversen V, Aimbire F and Lopes-Martins R A B 2006 Low-level laser therapy in acute pain: a systematic review of possible mechanisms of action and clinical effects in randomized placebo-controlled trials *Photomed. Laser Surg.* **24** 158–68

Bjordal J M, Lopes-Martins R A B, Joensen J, Coupp C, Ljunggren A E, Stergioulas A and Johnson M I 2008 A systematic review with procedural assessments and meta-analysis of low level laser therapy in lateral elbow tendinopathy (tennis elbow) *BMC Musculoskelet. Disord.* **9** 75

Boulnois J-L 1986 Photophysical processes in recent medical laser developments: a review. *Lasers Med. Sci.* **1** 47–66

Chow R T, Johnson M I, Lopes-Martins R A B and Bjordal J M 2009 Efficacy of low-level laser therapy in the management of neck pain: a systematic review and meta-analysis of randomised placebo or active-treatment controlled trials *Lancet* **374** 1897–908

Conlan M J, Rapley J W and Cobb C M 1996 Biostimulation of wound healing by low-energy laser irradiation—a review *J. Clin. Periodontol.* **23** 492–6

Duke D and Grevelink J M 1998 Care before and after laser skin resurfacing—a survey and review of the literature *Dermatol. Surg.* **24** 201–6

Hüttmann G, Yao C and Endl E 2005 New concepts in laser medicine: towards a laser surgery with cellular precision *Med. Laser Appl.* **20** 135–9

Kent K M and Graber E M 2012 Laser tattoo removal: a review *Dermatol. Surg.* **38** 1–13

Kimura Y, Wilder-Smith P and Matsumoto K 2000 Lasers in endodontics: a review *Int. Endod. J.* **33** 173–85

Kimura Y, Wilder-Smith P, Yonaga K and Matsumoto K 2000 Treatment of dentine hypersensitivity by lasers: a review *J. Clin. Periodontol.* **27** 715–21

Kitchen S S and Partridge C J 1991 A review of low level laser therapy part I: background, physiological effects and hazards *Physiotherapy* **77** 161–8

Langer D J and Vajkoczy O 2005 ELANA: Excimer laser-assisted nonocclusive anastomosis for extracranial-to-intracranial and intracranial-to-intracranial bypass: a review *Skull Base* **15** 191–205

Letokhov V S 1985 Laser biology and medicine *Nature* **316** 325–30

Martin T N, Knight D R, Ellison A G and Hillier V F 2004 Review of safety in endoscopic laser foraminoplasty for the management of back pain *J. Clin. Laser Med. Surg.* **19** 147–57

McKenzie A L 1990 Physics of thermal processes in laser-tissue interaction *Phys. Med. Biol.* **35** 1175–209
Mirhoseini M, Shelgikar S and Cayton M M 2009 Transmyocardial laser revascularization: a review *J. Clin. Laser Med. Surg.* **11** 15–9
Mundy L, Merlin T L, Fitridge R A and Hiller J E 2005 Systematic review of endovenous laser treatment for varicose veins *Br. J. Surg.* **92** 1189–94
Muqit M M K, Sanghvi C, McLauchlan R, Delgado C, Young L B, Charles S J, Marcellino G R and Stanga P E 2012 Study of clinical applications and safety for Pascal® laser photocoagulation in retinal vascular disorders *Acta Ophthalmol.* **90** 155–61
Parrish J A and Wilson B C 1991 Current and future trends in laser medicine *Photochem. Photobiol.* **53** 731–8
Peng Q, Juzeniene A, Chen J, Svaasand L O, Warloe T, Giercksky K-E and Moan J 2008 Lasers in medicine *Rep. Prog. Phys.* **71** 056701
Schindl A, Schindl M, Pernerstorfer-Schön H and Schindl L 2000 Low-intensity laser therapy: a review *J. Invest. Med.* **48** 312–26
Schwarz F, Aoki A, Becker J and Sculean A 2008 Laser application in non-surgical periodontal therapy: a systematic review *J. Clin. Periodontol.* **35** 29–44
Tumilty S, Munn J, McDonough S, Hurley D A, Basford J R and Baxter G D 2010 Low level laser treatment of tendinopathy: a systematic review with meta-analysis *Photomed. Laser Surg.* **28** 3–16
van Gemert M J C and Welch A J 1989 Time constants in thermal laser medicine *Lasers Surg. Med.* **9** 405–21
White J M, Chaudhry S I, Kudler J J, Sekandari N, Schoelch M L and Silverman S Jr 2009 Nd:YAG and CO_2 laser therapy of oral mucosal lesions *J. Clin. Laser Med. Surg.* **16** 299–304

www.ingramcontent.com/pod-product-compliance
Ingram Content Group UK Ltd.
Pitfield, Milton Keynes, MK11 3LW, UK
UKHW051853100926
8556IPUK00005B/605